Rethinking Hypothyroidism

RETHINHING HYPOTHYROIDISM

Why Treatment Must Change and
What Patients Can Do

ANTONIO C. BIANCO, MD

The University of Chicago Press
Chicago and London

The University of Chicago Press, Chicago 60637
The University of Chicago Press, Ltd., London
© 2022 by Antonio Bianco
Published 2022
Printed in the United States of America

31 30 29 28 27 26 25 24 23   2 3 4 5

ISBN-13: 978-0-226-82314-0 (cloth)
ISBN-13: 978-0-226-82316-4 (paper)
ISBN-13: 978-0-226-82315-7 (e-book)
DOI: https://doi.org/10.7208/chicago/9780226823157.001.0001

The information and suggestions contained in this book are not intended to replace the services of your physician or caregiver. Because each person and each medical situation is unique, you should consult your own physician to get answers to your personal questions, to evaluate any symptoms you may have, or to receive suggestions on appropriate medications.

The author has attempted to make this book as accurate and current as possible, but it may nevertheless contain errors, omissions, or material that is out of date at the time you read it. Neither the author nor the publisher have any legal responsibility or liability for errors, omissions, outdated material, or the reader's application of the medical information or advice contained in this book.

Library of Congress Cataloging-in-Publication Data

Names: Bianco, Antonio C., author.
Title: Rethinking hypothyroidism : why treatment must change and what patients can do / Antonio C. Bianco, MD.
Description: Chicago : University of Chicago Press, 2022. | Includes bibliographical references and index.
Identifiers: LCCN 2022017124 | ISBN 9780226823140 (cloth) | ISBN 9780226823164 (paperback) | ISBN 9780226823157 (ebook)
Subjects: LCSH: Hypothyroidism—Treatment.
Classification: LCC RC657 .B53 2022 | DDC 616.4/44—dc23/eng/20220610
LC record available at https://lccn.loc.gov/2022017124

To Laura, George, Michael, and Miriam

CONTENTS

PREFACE

Doctors commonly consider hypothyroidism an easy disease to treat. And yet, after years working as a physician and scientist, and as the former president of the American Thyroid Association, I could not square the fact that science had developed a successful treatment with the stories of some of my own patients, who continue to suffer.

They are not alone. For about 10–20% of patients on the leading treatment—millions in the United States and around the world—that treatment is not working. In this book, I argue that my fellow physicians need to take their patients' complaints seriously and give them more options. I arrive at this argument by explaining the details so that patients and their support networks can understand this complex subject and become their own advocates.

In the first part of the book, I cover the crisis that has evolved during the last fifty years, the role played by the pharmaceutical companies, and the dogmas and guidelines used by many doctors to justify ignoring their patients. In part 2 of the book, I provide the essential science necessary to understand why some of the recommendations in the guidelines are flawed. I have tried to make the science accessible to anyone interested, but patients most interested in treatment options might skip this part during a first reading without a major loss of understanding. In part 3, I review the history of hypothyroidism and its treatment, explaining our understanding as it developed over the past two hundred years. I have also tried to make this section accessible to all readers; again, though, patients might skip this section during a first reading if they want to understand treatment options more quickly.

Parts 1, 4, and 5 of the book are essential for all readers. Part 4 contains the scientific evidence supporting the claims made by millions of patients during the past fifty years. Patients will see confirmation that they are not alone and that their complaints have been shared and expressed for decades. In the final part of the book, I provide readers with specific information to help them understand alternative treatments for hypothyroidism. I also explain options for patients to discuss with their doctors that might reduce their symptoms. I end the book with a look at the future, with new technologies for improving the treatment of hypothyroidism.

I hope I have also provided enough detail for my secondary audience: my fellow physicians, medical students, and other healthcare professionals who care for patients with thyroid conditions. We all need to understand the problem and potential solutions and be part of the conversation. If a treatment isn't working for some, we can't call it a complete success.

For those who wish to gain in-depth knowledge of the disease mechanisms and clinical trials discussed in the book, I invite them to explore the references included in the book's citations and to visit PubMed (https://pubmed.ncbi.nlm.nih.gov/) using the obvious keywords and names of the scientists discussed in the book. I would also recommend visiting the websites of the American (https://www.thyroid.org/), British (https://www.british-thyroid-association.org/), and European (https://www.eurothyroid.com/) Thyroid Associations, as well as the British

Thyroid Foundation (https://www.btf-thyroid.org/). These sites contain vast amounts of specialized information. These are also useful for patients, as they contain additional practical advice and thoughtful lists of frequently asked questions, plus names and addresses of physicians who specialize in the treatment of thyroid disease. Please visit the BiancoLab website (http://deiodinase .org/) or follow me on Twitter (@Bianco_Lab) if you wish to know more about the work I do in my laboratory at the University of Chicago.

The treatment of hypothyroidism must change. Over the past five years, I have been thinking about this book, and I have spent the past two years writing it. I have decided to make my argument in the form of a story in which I describe my own research as well as hypothyroidism's long history and the science behind it. I learned how to do this when I was a teenager growing up in Brazil. My beloved aunt Rosinha would see me and immediately say, "Toninho, sit here and tell me a story." I do the same thing with my patients when we discuss their thyroid diseases. My hope is that my story, as told in this book, will give patients the tools they need to ultimately improve their own story.

Introduction

The story of hypothyroidism treatment presents a solution, followed by a mystery. Why did so many of those treated for hypothyroidism ultimately fare so poorly? How was a century-long
medical triumph transformed into a tarnished victory, fraught
with conflict and exhaustion? Why did doctors dismiss the millions of patients insisting their treatments were failing; and why
did patients find themselves suddenly doubting decades of reliable, tested science? How did the case of hypothyroidism back-
track from "closed" to "open"? Most important, what can these
patients who continue to suffer do? This book tells that story.

* * *

We start with the thyroid gland itself. There are several glands
in our body, and the thyroid is one of them. Glands typically
function by producing substances known as hormones that are
released into the bloodstream. These hormones travel through
the blood and reach distant organs, where they can regulate functions as diverse as blood levels of glucose, salt concentration, and
blood pressure.

First sketched as an organ by Leonardo da Vinci in the early
sixteenth century and named by the English physician Thomas

Wharton in 1656, the thyroid is a small gland located in the neck, right above the front of your shirt collar. It is shaped like a butterfly, weighs less than an ounce, and is not easily identified unless it is enlarged.

The thyroid gland takes up and concentrates the iodine that you normally ingest with meals and uses it to make thyroid hormones. The gland also releases into the circulation small amounts of its hormones throughout the day and night to regulate bodily functions. Additionally, it keeps a large storage of premade hormones that could sustain normal secretion for months, just in case you go through a period of reduced iodine intake.

Thyroid hormones affect virtually every organ in your body, accelerating the overall metabolism—your appetite and the rate at which you burn calories. These hormones also affect your memory, as well as the way you behave and think. Women will not become pregnant, and children will grow slowly or not at all without appropriate amounts of thyroid hormones. When the thyroid gland fails, a child may end up having a lower IQ and other neurological problems, and an adult will develop a disease known as hypothyroidism. Patients with hypothyroidism experience fatigue and sluggishness, sleep more than normal, have issues with the skin and hair, and gain weight.

In general, we physicians do a fairly good job at diagnosing hypothyroidism. The disease affects approximately five out of a hundred Americans, and hundreds of millions worldwide. Typically, hypothyroid patients have low levels of thyroid hormones in the circulation. Therefore, treatment is aimed at bringing these hormone levels back to typical levels. Treatment consists of daily supplemental doses of thyroid hormones taken by mouth, essentially complementing or even fully replacing the body production. Because hypothyroidism is so common, we likely know someone on thyroid-hormone supplementation—for example, levothyroxine, a.k.a. Synthroid, one of the popular brand names frequently prescribed to treat hypothyroidism.

While most patients with hypothyroidism who are treated with thyroid hormones do fairly well and see their doctors once every six to twelve months as recommended, a fraction of the patients treated for hypothyroidism (one and a half million to three million individuals in the United States) is far from living a normal life. Even though blood tests indicate their treatment is on target, these patients experience residual symptoms. They complain of what they call "foggy brain," mental confusion, difficulty making decisions, and poor memory. They also suffer from fatigue and difficulty managing body weight.

Unfortunately, physicians have been slow to recognize and treat these residual symptoms. In contrast to most patients doing well, there is a vocal minority truly suffering. The development of social media platforms accelerated the networking among patients that remain symptomatic. Dozens of patient-advocacy groups exist on multiple social media platforms, where patients voice their questions, frustrations, and anger toward physicians.

Major points of contention for patients include:

- How much of the standard thyroid hormone should be used in the treatment of hypothyroidism?
- Is it possible to add a second, more powerful thyroid hormone to the standard regimen?
- Should we employ a "natural treatment" made of thyroid extract, industrially prepared from animal thyroid and reduced to a powder?

Symptomatic patients and their doctors do have very different perspectives about these topics. Not surprisingly, the gap that was formed between us has been increasingly filled by individuals and entities that reportedly are there to help—but in many cases have emphasized the differences between doctors and patients and profited from alternative treatments, vitamins, diets, and other products.

* * *

I have been a scientist in the thyroid field and have seen patients with thyroid diseases for forty years. I run a laboratory funded by the National Institutes of Health (NIH) to study the mechanisms through which thyroid hormones regulate bodily functions. I have also had many patients with hypothyroidism who were members of that unfortunate minority who could not return to normal life—despite getting standard treatment, as well as passing all the thyroid tests that I was trained to provide. But up until the early 2010s, I was oblivious to the magnitude of this problem. As I became more involved with these patients of mine, I learned they were not alone.

Their impact on me led me to refocus my research toward understanding why they were suffering—and, more important, how this problem could be fixed. In the last decade, I have published several studies that have helped identify the problem and the reasons some patients with hypothyroidism on thyroid-hormone supplementation could have residual symptoms. In addition, my studies shed light on how residual symptoms develop. I have also joined forces with other scientists around the world and consulted for several pharmaceutical companies to help develop new forms of treatment for hypothyroidism. My goal is to improve the quality of life of all patients with hypothyroidism.

* * *

What scientists have learned over the last century about the thyroid gland is fascinating, and their efforts have resulted in two

Nobel Prizes in Physiology or Medicine. The Swiss surgeon Theodor Kocher received the Nobel Prize in 1909 for his work on the physiology, pathology, and surgery of the thyroid gland; in 1977, two neuroscientists, the French American Roger Guillemin and the Lithuanian American Andrew V. Schally split half the prize for their discoveries of how the brain controls thyroid function.

Our story starts at the turn of the nineteenth century, when endemic goiter (an enlargement of the thyroid) and what was called cretinism (an irreversible developmental delay caused by congenital or neonatal hypothyroidism) were common and scientists were studying the possible connection between both. Later, those investigating the gland realized that a healthy thyroid gland secretes hormones that affect every aspect of the body. Thus, the disease hypothyroidism occurs whenever the thyroid gland is not working or is surgically removed, and consequently, the levels of these hormones in the blood drop below normal range. Low levels of thyroid hormones are what cause the well-known symptoms related to hypothyroidism.

To reverse these symptoms, patients in those early days were treated with extracts of the thyroid gland obtained from sheep, cows, or pigs. This approach was developed in the 1890s and lasted through the better part of the twentieth century. The extracts contained a mixture of hormones that hypothyroid patients couldn't produce on their own, later known as T_4 and T_3, each a collection of four or three iodine atoms, respectively.

Today's conventional treatment for hypothyroidism also aims at normalizing the circulating levels of these hormones. However, it does so with only one of these crucial hormones, T_4, created in a laboratory and administered at a precise dosage. What is the rationale for replacing a mixture of T_4 and T_3 with only T_4? After absorption into the bloodstream, your body transforms T_4 into T_3, the main active hormone that resolves the symptoms of hypothyroidism.

It was only after the standard of care became treatment with T_4 only that we see reports of dissatisfaction by fully treated patients with hypothyroidism. At the time this change in the approach to treat hypothyroidism was happening, many patients complained as they were being switched to therapy with T_4. Based on interviews with my colleagues who were treating patients in the 1960s and 1970s, approximately one-quarter of the patients placed on T_4 requested to return to thyroid extract or did not switch at all. Nonetheless, the switch moved forward unabated, and today, T_4 is among the top prescription medicines in the United States, with annual sales of billions of dollars worldwide.

In retrospect, I can't help but wonder why most of us ignored these early warnings and so easily wrote off patients' complaints without questioning the effectiveness of T_4. How this happened is a fascinating story that evolved over the last two hundred years, with all the ingredients of an exciting drama. It involves an incapacitating disease that predominantly affects women; an effective low-tech treatment (thyroid extract) that had potency problems and was vilified and abandoned in favor of a lucrative synthetic molecule; top-notch medical research and discoveries that backed up this new treatment and swayed medical opinion; a culture of patient dismissal; and, of course, money and pharmaceutical influence.

This is the story of hypothyroidism. And it is the story of this book.

PART ONE

The Crisis

CHAPTER 1

Treatments and Controversies

Dear Dr. Bianco,

I know my body well enough to know when the thyroid is out of sorts. I had a sense of being unwell this entire season. Before my college classes start in the fall, I must get regulated. I am the type of person who never misses a day of work. I believe this crisis is the result of a doctor taking me off of thyroid extract and not giving me T_3. He just gave me T_4 . . . I cannot walk a straight line and am in a constant state of dizziness. My vision is blurry and I feel like I have vertigo. I have chronic insomnia and am extremely jumpy. I cannot focus and worse of all cannot focus on reading. My thyroid problems all started when the brand I was taking of thyroid extract went off the market. Since then I have had a 30-pound weight gain. I cannot understand why all these new meds cannot do the job of that thyroid extract. I think this drug was taken off the market several times . . . each time when I go back on it, I feel healthy and have the energy and alertness of a 20-year-old. Would you please give me both T_4 and T_3?

Emails like this were pouring into my inbox in the summer of 2011. My clinic at the University of Miami was packed with pa-tients having hypothyroidism. Patients with hypothyroidism are knowledgeable about their condition. They know that it can be caused by thyroid surgery, but the overwhelming majority have Hashimoto's disease. This is an autoimmune condition in which the body produces antibodies and activates cells to destroy the thyroid gland.

Those emails got me concerned because they indicated that the number of treated yet dissatisfied patients with hypothyroidism was increasing.

This was not entirely new. This trend had started four decades previously, following a couple of modifications that thyroid experts had made to the way patients are treated. They introduced these changes almost all at the same time. The changes were logical and well meaning, so the complaints that followed caught physicians off guard. After all, clinician-scientists had developed effective treatment for hypothyroidism in the 1890s, and physicians had been making use of it without much fail since then. By all accounts, the changes introduced were commonsensical, based on science, and intended to make a good treatment even better.

In comparison with other chronic diseases, the strategy to treat hypothyroidism is slightly different. For example, when a patient suffers from heart failure (inability of the heart to pump sufficient blood), we first try to understand what is affecting the heart, and, if it is treatable, to use the appropriate medical or surgical procedure to fix the problem. We also use drugs that can either strengthen the heart muscle or lower the resistance against which blood is pumped, making it easier for blood to flow. Either way, the goal is to heal the heart.

In the case of hypothyroidism, we do not treat the thyroid. We forget about the thyroid, which no longer works or simply has been surgically removed. Instead, we supply the body with the amounts of thyroid hormones that would normally be secreted into the circulation by a healthy thyroid. If this is done correctly, the body will not know the difference and the patient can return to having a normal life.

If not treated, hypothyroidism can be incapacitating, with serious decrements of the quality of life, mental and physical sluggishness, constipation, a loss of appetite, a hoarse voice, leg cramps, cold intolerance, and weight gain. Over time, patients who are not treated can also suffer from hair loss and see a change in their appearances, such as a broadened nose, swollen lips and tongue, swollen eyelids, and brittle nails. Their skin can become pale, cool, and waxy, and exhibit a yellowish discoloration. Fortunately, supplementation with thyroid hormones resolves these symptoms. And thus, when some patients started to experience symptoms of hypothyroidism despite the new treatment, they were puzzled but felt confident physicians could fix their problem.

Physicians seemed to be on top of things. They understood how the thyroid gland works and had been treating patients with hypothyroidism for many decades. Treatment was solid, a no-brainer. For example, in the 1960s, backed by seventy years of experience, physicians considered that, when properly managed, treatment with thyroid extract—a crude preparation of animal thyroid in which the thyroid gland from pigs is reduced to a powder and packaged in tablets—reproduced the effects of natural thyroid secretion without toxicity.

Indeed, the top thyroid physicians at the Thyroid Unit at the Massachusetts General Hospital at Harvard Medical School in Boston, James Means, Leslie DeGroot, and John Stanbury, stated in their 1963 book, *The Thyroid and Its Diseases*, that "a diagnosis of hypothyroidism having been made [in an uncomplicated patient] the next logical step is to give thyroid [extract]. The results that follow such treatment are prompt and dramatic. They are of scientific as well as practical interest."[1]

Of course, we now know that most of those patients were being overtreated, which is definitively not good—probably a time bomb, given the long-term consequences to the heart and bones. But the quote above helps us get situated and understand the state of mind of most physicians at that time.

The newly introduced changes of the 1970s called for treatment with a synthetic molecule of T_4—the main hormone secreted by the thyroid—at doses adjusted based on the circulating levels of what is called thyroid-stimulating hormone, or TSH. Measuring TSH blood levels is the current gold standard for the diagnosis of hypothyroidism.

TSH is secreted into the circulation by the pituitary gland, which is connected to the brain. Together, these organs constantly measure the levels of thyroid hormones in the circulation and respond by adjusting the TSH secretion. TSH is a hormone that stimulates the thyroid to function. Thus, it makes sense that TSH levels are elevated when thyroid-hormone levels are low. An elevated TSH stimulates the thyroid to secrete more thyroid hormones, which will then restore levels to normal. This method to adjust the dose of T_4 made sense because TSH levels are elevated in the blood of hypothyroid patients and promptly return to normal upon treatment.

With these changes between the 1970s and 1980s, more and more patients with hypothyroidism found themselves complaining of residual symptoms. While they were adequately treated for hypothyroidism under the new approach, some of their symptoms remained.

Patients complained to their physicians as early as 1970.[2] However, the medical establishment's enthusiasm for the synthetic T_4 was high, and nothing of substance was done to clarify the issue of residual symptoms. It was only twenty-six years later, in 1996, that patients went on record and registered their frustration. Prompted by a clinical psychologist who was alarmed at the increasing number of patients with unresolved thyroid-related symptoms, patients in the United Kingdom wrote dozens of letters expressing their frustration over lingering symptoms.[3] They not only complained about residual symptoms but also of their doctors. They complained of a lack of empathy and instead receiving referrals to psychiatrists. Twenty-five years later, things had not gotten any better. Frustration with treatment for hypothyroidism is now a worldwide phenomenon. Patients continue to share and express similar feelings, as illustrated in this patient's message I received in the spring of 2020:

> I was diagnosed hypothyroid fifteen years ago. Following that diagnosis, for the reasons you mentioned, finding treatment that was effective for and acceptable to me was difficult as the four doctors and endocrinologists I visited just didn't listen and wouldn't talk with me. There was an established treatment; do it and we don't want to talk about it. I distinctly remember an endocrinologist I visited to discuss the questions I had after doing my research and he leaned over, patted my knee and said, "You let me worry about all that, dear." So much for doctor/patient collaboration.

* * *

In 2016, the American Thyroid Association asked Jacqueline (Jacquie) Jonklaas, a clinician-scientist at Georgetown University in Washington, DC, and me to organize and cochair a symposium on hypothyroidism. We had organized symposia many times, but this time we wanted to innovate and bring patients' perspectives into the discussion. We asked colleagues with expertise in hypothyroidism to join our effort and formed a committee to guarantee that a variety of views and perspectives were showcased at the symposium. After a few conference calls to discuss the program, we settled on adopting two ideas.

The committee would create an online survey for patients with hypothyroidism that would, for the first time, couple real numbers to the perspectives of patients with hypothyroidism. This data could then be presented during the symposium. We would also invite patients to participate in the symposium to voice their ideas and concerns and debate openly with the physicians. There were discussions and some resistance about a live debate with patients. Physicians are not used to this; I heard, "We can only invite patients we trust." Nonetheless, we moved forward, prepared the survey, and invited the patients.

The online survey remained open for a little more than a month. It was publicized among patient groups but not on major news outlets. The results were unprecedented—unexpected.[4] About 10,500 women and five hundred men with hypothyroidism completed the survey, figures which reflected the 9:1 ratio by which hypothyroidism affects women and men. The results revealed a great deal of dissatisfaction among patients.

On a scale of 0 to 10 (10 being the maximum), patients returned a median score of 5 to 6 when asked about their satisfaction level with treatment. We were surprised to see that they also returned a score of 5 to 6 when asked about their current physicians. Patients revealed that they had changed physicians multiple times, some up to ten times.

When asked to indicate the relevant areas they felt were not resolved by thyroid-hormone supplementation, most cited "fatigue," "memory," and "weight management." They returned a median score of 10 when asked about life disruption and the need for new treatments. The live testimonial provided by two patients was emotional and reflected the information collected online.

*   *   *

Brain fog is one of the residual symptoms mentioned in the survey, and one that I frequently hear of from symptomatic patients on T_4. This is an unspecified condition that thyroid doctors do not normally consider a symptom. We physicians are not even sure what it means. Patients with several other diseases and conditions—including cancer treatment, celiac disease, chronic fatigue syndrome, COVID-19, and lupus—complain of brain fog. But, what do T_4-treated patients mean when they say they have brain fog?

To approach this question I brought in Miriam Ribeiro, a scientist at MacKenzie Presbyterian University in São Paulo, Brazil, and a former fellow of mine, who specializes in endocrine regulation of cognitive functions. We decided to create a survey, but this time aimed at patients with hypothyroidism currently under treatment and experiencing brain fog. We asked Matt Ettleson, a clinical fellow in my group, to lead the survey. He worked with experts in the field and put together an online survey, which remained open for about one month in the winter of 2020; it received about 5,500 responses. Patients described four chief symptoms: fatigue, feeling sleepy, mental confusion, and difficulty focusing. These symptoms were present most of the day.

I would not have thought that brain fog and fatigue could be linked. The connection is not intuitive. But there could be an explanation. Many of our daily activities demand attention. To sustain a reasonable level of focused attention, you need to gate competing stimuli or thoughts so that you can pay attention to one at a time. The constant demand of this inhibitory control over diverse stimuli ends up depleting focused attention, and the result is fatigue.

In one of the questions, we asked patients what they did to feel better. Ava Raine, an undergraduate student working with Ettleson, compiled their responses, finding that about half cited behavior modifications such as resting or exercising, as well as a good diet, more caffeine, and less work-related stress (5–10% each). Fifteen percent of the patients also mentioned that adjusting the dose of thyroid hormones was important, and 10% mentioned that T_3—the other thyroid hormone, more potent than T_4—or thyroid extract improved symptoms.

The survey also contained an open field where participants could write anything they thought was important. About 2,500 patients did. Their comments were jaw dropping. Alice Batistuzzo and Samuel Batista, two of Ribeiro's graduate students, together with Maria Cristina Teixeira, also a scientist at MacKenzie Presbyterian University, studied their responses using a textual data-analysis software developed in collaboration with the National Center for Scientific Research in France. The analysis identified groups of patients that were focused on four different things.

- Cognitive issues (memory problems—about 40%—and mental confusion—about 10%)
- The poor doctor-patient relationship (about 20%)
- The burden of carrying a lifelong chronic condition (about 15%)
- Adjustments of their medication (about 15%)

While we are just learning about these subcategories, it would be amazing if doctors tried to match their own patients with one of these four subcategories, so that they could address patient concerns in a more focused way.

It was striking to see what patients said about their definition of brain fog: "makes me feel dumb and ineffective," "hinders my ability to find the right word," "a veil of fatigue comes over entirety," "a dream state but you are awake," "severe fatigue and feels like I am walking through sludge," "cloud of nothing in my brain," "it is like your brain is in static," "a constant feeling of wired and tired, fatigue and angst, exhaustion, and restlessness," "you constantly feel like a zombie," "if you are not a smoker, go smoke a cigarette and give it five minutes—this is my best way to describe it." They also mentioned how deeply brain fog affected their professional lives.

*   *   *

According to patients, since 1970, physicians have used a cookie-cutter approach to treat hypothyroidism: prescribe daily tablets of T_4 at doses that normalize TSH levels and that's it. Physicians explain that normal TSH levels indicate that the dose of T_4 is adequate and there is nothing else that should be done. This is illustrated in the following email:

> I have been bounced all over . . . by mainstream doctors who say "TSH is all that matters" and "we only prescribe Synthroid until your TSH falls in range regardless of symptoms." Can you please help me with a different view? Thank you.

This approach led those symptomatic patients to complain that looking to TSH levels when adjusting the dose of T_4 is just plain wrong. I heard this from many of my patients. The phrase "TSH levels do not matter. I know my body" became famous. It has been used many times by patients and, sadly, as a joke among physicians—even present in "satirical" YouTube videos ridiculing patients' insistence on the residual symptoms.[5]

One way some patients alleviate their residual symptoms is by ignoring TSH levels and increasing their dose of T_4 on their own. Indeed, there have been countless times when I have seen patients who were overtreated with T_4. Their TSH levels were too low, sometimes undetectable—an indication that the dose of T_4 is too high. Frequently, as I would explain the need to reduce their dose of T_4 because of possible dangerous consequences to the heart and bones—increased risk of atrial fibrillation and osteoporosis—patients would stop me and throw the cookie-cutter approach right back at me. "You just care about TSH levels and not how we really feel," they would say.

Others alleviate their symptoms through the use of combination therapy, a combination of two tablets, T_4 + T_3. A popular brand name of T_3 is Cytomel. Some patients even go a step further: they abandon synthetic forms of thyroid hormones altogether and look instead to thyroid extract (several brands are available), which contains both T_4 and T_3. Earlier in my career, I tried to persuade these patients to abandon combination therapy or thyroid extract in favor of T_4 alone. The training that I had received and the clinical guidelines I followed served as my professional guidance. These informed me of one thing: the new treatment, T_4, was and continues to be the standard of care. Indeed, treatment with T_4 worked for most patients.

I was skeptical about thyroid extract as well as the combination therapy T_4 + T_3. I assumed thyroid extract was unreliable, and no studies showed the long-term safety of any type of combination therapy. Neither was superior to T_4 alone. Frankly, I said these things to my patients without knowing all the facts. I was just repeating what I learned—that is, to be skeptical of combination therapy, and only vaguely knowledgeable about what thyroid extract is.

Some patients would just say thank you, and never come back. Others would respond with something like, "Dr. Bianco, I thought you were different," or "You're part of the TSH mafia," or "I had this discussion with my previous doctors and I know that if I reduce the dose of T_4 [or stop taking T_3 or thyroid extract], I won't feel well," or "I know my body, I know what I need, I cannot live with a normal TSH level or without T_3 or thyroid extract."

Before I became aware of the controversies surrounding therapy for hypothyroidism, I would just dismiss these complaints and renew the prescription with what I thought was an appropriate dose of T_4; I would not renew a prescription for T_3 or thyroid extract, to the frustration of many.

But this approach led to so much pushback from patients that, with time, I started handling it differently. I learned that listening takes you a long way with these patients. So, I would listen, be sympathetic, and try to talk patients into a compromise, laying out a plan through which their dose of T_4 would be reduced over time or, as with T_3 and thyroid extract, switched off entirely.

I lost most battles but, in the process, I believe I helped many patients. While in many cases I was able to reduce the dose of T_4 and bring TSH levels up to normal, I cannot recall a single patient that I successfully convinced to stop taking either T_3 or thyroid extract. Patients would go back and forth with doses of both medications, never to be on T_4 alone. As I said, in many cases, the patients would never return. They would just go see a different physician to try getting a prescription containing T_3 or thyroid extract.

*   *   *

My approach to symptomatic patients with hypothyroidism, which in retrospect seems insensitive, was not unique. Many physicians used a similar approach across the country and, of course, conspiracy theories developed. Most patients could not understand—and still can't—why we were or are unwilling to prescribe combination therapy or thyroid extract if these regimens made them feel better.

Some patient-advocacy groups claimed physicians were influenced by the pharmaceutical companies to just prescribe T_4. A quick search on the internet identifies a series of articles, blogs, and chat rooms pointing to conspiracy theories about T_4. This is a sample of what can be found online:

We ARE wary of guidelines that implicitly establish partnerships between pharmaceuticals and medical professionals by assuming every hypothyroid patient is currently taking T_4 or should be. Mass persuasion to prescribe one medication alone has rigged the marketplace and limited choice and awareness of diversity. This system has unfairly established and entrenched T_4 monotherapy's dominance over all thyroid therapy.[6]

Feeling unassisted by their doctors, patients did what little they could do, which was to organize around advocacy groups. As one can imagine, social media accelerated networking among these patients. They connected and strengthened their voices. Today, there are dozens of patient-advocacy groups with hundreds of thousands of members organized around the theme of hypothyroidism and residual symptoms during treatment with T_4. The main idea is to exchange experiences and information, which is a very laudable goal.

In the United States and around the world, several patient-based top-notch organizations support patients with thyroid diseases. The British Thyroid Foundation is an example of a phenomenal group that advocates on behalf of patients, with particular effort on hypothyroidism. They are a group of volunteers who built a network of telephone contacts, local groups, and Facebook groups, to offer support based on patient experience. Their work on prescriptions for T_3 illustrates their strength. As we will see throughout this book, many dissatisfied patients with hypothyroidism report that combination therapy ($T_4 + T_3$) makes them feel better. However, over the last few years, many patients in the United Kingdom have found that obtaining a prescription for T_3 has become difficult. Medicine in the United Kingdom is highly socialized, and local health budgets are controlled by clinical commissioning groups. These groups have generally adopted a very strict line toward the treatment of hypothyroidism, and this has impacted both the patients who have been stable on T_3 for many years (many of whom appear to have had their prescriptions withdrawn abruptly) and also those who don't feel well on T_4 and may benefit from a trial of combination therapy.

Consequently, I learned from my colleague Peter Taylor, a clinician-scientist in Cardiff, Wales, that to remain on T_3, a patient in the United Kingdom must pay out of pocket for an endocrinologist who agrees to prescribe and provide follow-up, as well as for the medication. The estimated price of T_3 in the United Kingdom is $2,700 per patient per year! However, thanks to the work of the British Thyroid Foundation and local patient-advocacy groups in Norfolk and Waveney, the regional committee created a "T_3 Commissioning Pathway" that rationalizes the prescription of T_3 for patients with hypothyroidism, hoping that the protocol may be adopted more widely.

*　*　*

Unfortunately, some group organizers also came to the debate with ulterior motives, be it to sell advice books, peddle dietary supplements, provide obscure certifications, or otherwise without any evidence or scientific rationale to back up their claims. The influence of these groups through social media was huge. Naturally, they did all this while also criticizing the physicians. These groups occupy an existing niche between patients with hypothyroidism and their physicians; hence, the greater the distance between the two, the better their chances are to prevail in peddling their claims.

This animus irritated many physicians, who concluded unfairly that, in reaching out to symptomatic patients, they would be "giving in" to those groups critical of the physicians. I've tried to discuss this situation with my colleagues numerous times; however, most have decided to ignore anything relating to patients on T_4 with residual symptoms precisely because of these organizations. For them, it might otherwise be too frustrating to deal with the disruptive and negative influence attributed to these groups, which they mistakenly believe to be inherent in working with patients suffering from residual symptoms. Once, while meeting with my colleagues, I proposed reaching out to patients with hypothyroidism to establish a mutually beneficial relationship. They looked at one another and, after a few seconds, laughed.

This situation has persisted for years. The lack of concern among physician leadership and professional societies strikes me as remarkable. They have simply dismissed any criticism, labeling it as unfounded and not worthy of a response. Acknowledgment that some patients with hypothyroidism remain symptomatic is seen as giving credence to the individuals who benefit from the problem—those who accuse physicians of being insensitive and manipulated by pharmaceutical companies.

Such a rigid position is indeed unexpected, given that professional societies are well organized around groups of patients with other thyroid diseases—patients with Graves' disease (a form of hyperthyroidism), patients with thyroid cancer, and others. In fact, in these cases, this is so well organized that, not infrequently, these groups campaign for funds earmarked for research in partnership with thyroid societies.

Using these successful models, we could have created bridges with serious patient-advocacy groups formed by patients with hypothyroidism. This would have signaled to patients that we want to listen and try to understand the problem. We could have included patient leaders to establish communication channels, develop and implement a plan of action.

As far as I know, nothing like that was ever tried for patients with hypothyroidism. There has been no consistent attempt to directly reach out to groups of patients with hypothyroidism in the United States. We kept missing the opportunity to bridge those gaps. So, physicians and patients have continued to grow further apart for decades. This is ironic: hypothyroidism is the disease that by far channeled the most support from pharmaceutical companies to physicians, scientists, and professional societies, and yet we have not fostered a productive relationship with affected patients.

* * *

My thyroid clinics at the University of Miami were on Monday mornings—one of the high points of my week. The staff was great, always cheerful, and helpful. I loved it because it was my chance to talk to the patients, many of whom spoke Spanish. The clinic was always busy, but I took my time and chatted with everybody about their families, their native countries, their work, food, and of course, their thyroids.

About a quarter of my patients were from Cuba, and much to my surprise, many had arrived only a few months earlier. Some patients brought handwritten notes in wrapping paper from Cuba, containing lab results or prescriptions, sometimes even pills in small paper bags. They were good people, and we laughed a lot. After ten years of working in Boston, I welcomed familiar faces and cultures that reminded me of my native country of Brazil.

In the beginning, I must admit, the language barrier was a challenge. Even though Portuguese and Spanish are grammatically similar, they sound very different, and Brazilians do not regularly learn Spanish as a second language. Nonetheless, I was also no stranger to the language. I had sort of gotten used to Spanish during the 1980s, after years of learning and working during medical school with Carlos Roberto Douglas, a Chilean expat who fled the Pinochet regime and directed the Physiology Department at Santa Casa School of Medicine in São Paulo, where I graduated from.

In Miami, I dusted off my Spanish; if things got complicated at the clinic, I could always rely on one of the medical assistants for help, as many of them were native speakers. At the clinics, I had colleagues from different specialties who could discuss and plan for the tough cases right then and there. Having the surgeons around streamlined treatment and made it easier for my patients, most of whom had thyroid cancer. For the most part, such cases require thyroid surgery, an operation that nearly always leads to hypothyroidism. I also had plenty of patients who developed hypothyroidism due to Hashimoto's disease. I have seen thousands of patients with thyroid disease throughout my career. However, as I will explain, hypothyroidism in particular first drew my attention in this clinic after seeing two patients, weeks apart, but with very similar stories (more on this later).

In general, my routine with patients with hypothyroidism was simple enough. Patients frequently came to my office on the referral of other physicians, because a screening blood test during checkup had found elevated TSH levels. Indeed, this is how most cases of hypothyroidism are diagnosed everywhere. While the normal reference range for TSH is 0.45 to 4.5 microunits per milliliter (μU/ml), TSH levels that are higher than 10 μU/ml strongly indicate hypothyroidism. Values between 5 and 10 μU/ml could indicate thyroid problems but require further considerations. In addition, there are cases in which the diagnosis of hypothyroidism can be anticipated—for example, after most of the thyroid gland is removed through surgery, or after treatment with radioactive iodine. In the case of surgery, treatment can start upon hospital discharge, even before abnormal TSH levels are detected.

Signs and symptoms assist in the diagnosis of hypothyroidism. However, a diagnosis cannot be established without those blood tests. Many patients, encouraged by people not familiar with hypothyroidism, measure basal body temperature first thing in the morning to self-diagnose hypothyroidism. While a lower body temperature might be a sign of an obvious case of hypothyroidism, also known as overt hypothyroidism, this approach lacks the sensitivity and specificity necessary to be used as a faithful diagnostic tool. One area of intense research is the search for a blood marker that could be used in association with or to replace TSH. Biomarkers, as these molecules are called, are often thought of as an alternative for detecting hypothyroidism, but they are not sufficiently developed at the moment to be used outside of a research context.

So, upon seeing those patients at the clinic, my approach was to confirm the elevation in blood TSH from their checkup by obtaining a new TSH measure as well as the levels of thyroid hormones (which could be reduced to below normal). Recall that the elevation in TSH blood levels seen in patients with hypothyroidism is meant to stimulate the thyroid gland to secrete more hormones. However, either these patients did not have a thyroid gland, or their thyroid wasn't functioning properly and couldn't respond to TSH stimulation.

So, I would prescribe the standard treatment, which was to supplement the inadequate levels of thyroid hormones with T_4 tablets, at doses that made the TSH levels return to the normal reference range. I would make sure the TSH levels normalized after a few months, and send the patients back to their primary doctor with a "thank you for your referral" letter. According to the most respected models, such a process was wholly unremarkable. It was an example of the successful care that modern medicine provided, addressing a disease known and treated for over a century.

Other patients were referred to me because they were women having difficulty becoming pregnant—and with a questionable

TSH level—or women with established hypothyroidism who became pregnant and needed a thyroid doctor to oversee their treatment during pregnancy. Thyroid hormones are important for fertility and a healthy pregnancy. During pregnancy, the placenta accelerates the metabolism of T_4 and T_3 to minimize the amount of maternal thyroid hormones that the fetus receives. In response, a woman with a healthy thyroid gland will simply accelerate the secretion of thyroid hormones and in many cases develop a visible goiter during pregnancy, which returns to normal after delivery. But this possibility is not available for someone with hypothyroidism because the thyroid does not function well or has been removed. Thus, immediately upon learning of a new pregnancy, doctors orient women with hypothyroidism to increase the dose of T_4 by about 30% (one to two extra tablets per week) to counteract the accelerated placental destruction of thyroid hormones. Not doing so will expose the developing fetus to lower thyroid-hormone levels, which could have disastrous consequences, such as a child with a lower IQ.

*   *   *

Yet at other times, patients with hypothyroidism came to my office because, despite treatment with T_4 and a normal TSH level, they continued to experience hypothyroidism symptoms. In this case, I would confirm their diagnosis and that the dose of T_4 was right for them. In some cases, the dose was off, and, by adjusting it, the patients would feel better. I would also look for other diseases or conditions that could explain their "residual" symptoms.

If nothing that could explain the symptoms was found, I would tell the patients that the residual symptoms were not thyroid related. I would not question the new treatment developed in the 1970s. Instead—I now regret to admit—I would recommend the patient see a psychotherapist. What else could explain the residual symptoms?

But this routine changed after I met the two remarkable patients. I saw them a few weeks apart, and what struck me about them was that they were both middle-aged teachers. Both of them, from Cuban areas in or outside Miami, had left their jobs only months after being diagnosed with hypothyroidism, despite treatment with T_4.

One patient underwent surgical thyroidectomy (removal of the thyroid gland) for thyroid nodules. A thyroidectomy can be partial, in which case there is a chance that the residual thyroid fragment will increase production and sustain normal thyroid secretion without the need for supplementation with T_4. However, my patient had a total thyroidectomy. She stayed in the hospital for two days and was immediately placed on T_4. This is a very common surgery performed by endocrine surgeons as well as ear-nose-and-throat (ENT) surgeons. Conservative estimates suggest that about 150,000 thyroidectomies are performed each year in the United States. In general, a thyroidectomy is very safe, but in a very small number of cases, there could be complications with the vocal cords and other neighboring glands, depending on the surgeon's skill and on the severity of the thyroid disease itself.

My patient told me that, right from the start, she felt off. A dynamic middle school math teacher before the surgery, she found it increasingly difficult to fall back into that lifestyle following her treatment. The other patient was not different. She was a very active high school teacher who slowly lost her ability to focus and keep up with her busy schedule and multitasking. She saw a doctor who diagnosed her with hypothyroidism and immediately placed her on T_4. She also never returned to how she had been before her diagnosis.

These teachers had become unfocused and lethargic, and had

gained weight. Their treatment plans were adequate according to guidelines, and blood tests indicated both were taking the correct dosage of T_4. Everything indicated that they should have felt fine, but they did not. They both felt extremely unhappy and left their careers out of frustration, shame, and sadness, as well as respect for their students.

I followed my routine. After I investigated the possibility of other conditions and failed to find anything, I recommended that the first patient see a psychotherapist. She was distressed and cried. Her husband, who was also in the room, was visibly upset. They had heard that I was a thyroid doctor from Harvard and had hoped I could help.

When I heard such a similar story from the second patient, I realized something was wrong. For the first time, I saw that the way we, physicians, understood hypothyroidism—a disease for which we allegedly had developed an effective treatment— needed a new direction. For this patient, I did venture out of my routine and offered combination therapy for hypothyroidism for the first time in my life. The year was 2011. A few weeks later, she called me to say how grateful she was. She had improved substantially, "as if a fog veil had been lifted from my mind," she said. I called the first patient and placed her on the same regimen with T_3. Unfortunately, I never heard from her again.

*   *   *

As I acquired more experience with symptomatic patients on T_4 and talked to colleagues who also saw these patients, it became clear to me that in many cases the thyroid gland (or hypothyroidism) was not to blame. To start, not all patients placed on T_4 have a formal diagnosis of hypothyroidism, which complicates the investigation and treatment of true residual symptoms. Physicians have different thresholds to place patients on T_4. The relative ease with which this happens is driven by the perceived idea that T_4 is safe, as well as by patients who are convinced they have hypothyroidism and demand treatment.

The drive to place patients on T_4 is intense. Physicians are bombarded with the message, in different formats, that T_4 is not only fully effective but also safe—so much so that, when in doubt as to whether a patient even has hypothyroidism, many physicians tend to prescribe T_4 anyway. The patients come to us with a frustrating complaint and expect a diagnosis and treatment. In some cases, there is clear pressure from the patients to give out a prescription, and some of us do fold to it.

This is how it happens. The main symptoms of hypothyroidism—fatigue, weight gain, and impaired cognition—can be caused by many conditions. Other chronic conditions, such as anemia, diabetes, heart failure, and certain vitamin deficiencies, may mimic residual symptoms or can complicate the management of hypothyroidism. Thus, patients with suggestive symptoms and a TSH level in the upper limit of normal end up being placed on T_4.

Consider a forty-five-year-old female patient I saw in Miami. She suffered from symptoms that are typical of hypothyroidism, such as low energy, dry skin, cold intolerance, and constipation. However, her TSH levels upon diagnosis were within normal range, albeit in the upper limit of normal, 3.7 µU/ml (normal range in most cases is 0.45 to 4.5 µU/ml). While national and international guidelines do not support treatment for such a patient, her previous physician started her on T_4 without further testing or findings that would have supported a diagnosis of hypothyroidism.

By placing this patient on T_4, her former doctor labeled her as having hypothyroidism for the rest of her life, when, in fact, she does not. Subsequently, any future symptoms this patient might develop would be automatically pinned on her nonexistent hypothyroidism. Indeed, she came to see me because her treatment with T_4 wasn't working. I would have been surprised if it did, as the baseline TSH was normal (which means she did not have hypothyroidism). In my Miami practice, probably once a month I would take a patient off T_4, because they had been started on the drug without a proper diagnosis of hypothyroidism.

It was the same story when I moved to Chicago. A few years ago, I saw a patient who an acquaintance had recommended to me, who had absolutely no reason to be on T_4. When informed that she should not have been on T_4, she got frustrated and rapidly left my office.

This phenomenon seems to be widespread. A collaborative project conducted by several groups in the United States analyzed about 1,100 patients (86% women) being treated with T_4.[7] Treatment for all patients was suspended, and the patients were reassessed for hypothyroidism. A staggering one-third of the patients were found to have normal thyroid function, even after T_4 was suspended.

Another group of symptomatic patients consists of individuals previously diagnosed and treated for hypothyroidism, resolving their symptoms. Years later, they relapse and become symptomatic again. Hypothyroidism is so frequent that it is common to see an association between it and other chronic conditions. Menopausal syndrome is a typical example of this association: hypothyroidism is common in women and all women go through menopause. The symptoms are indeed very similar. I was fortunate that many years ago I recruited Jennifer Glueck, a physician and graduate of the Endocrinology Fellowship at the University of Miami who specializes in female reproductive endocrinology and menopausal syndrome, to join the division. Many of my T_4-treated patients with hypothyroidism with normal TSH levels who develop symptoms years later were going through menopausal syndrome and benefited greatly from seeing Glueck and, when appropriate, initiating estrogen replacement therapy.

In my experience and that of my colleagues, it has always been helpful to pinpoint when residual symptoms started. I interpret symptoms that start around the time of diagnosis and continue while on T_4 as indicative of symptoms of hypothyroidism that respond partially to T_4. In contrast, if the symptoms started years before or years after, it is unlikely to reflect a shortcoming of T_4 treatment.

If, after considering all this, I cannot find alternative explanations for the residual symptoms, I assume that a patient unequivocally did not fully benefit from treatment with T_4. There is no roadmap for what to do next. On their own, as we have seen, patients will pursue lifestyle modifications. A minority of physicians will attempt combination therapy. Others will prescribe thyroid extract, falling back on a practice developed in the 1890s. One thing is clear: if we can't help a patient—and in some cases, we can't—they will move on to a new endocrinologist, repeat a large series of tests, and perhaps go through a similar process.

This cycle will repeat itself multiple times until patients grow too tired of moving around or find a health professional who is able to address their frustrations. The survey we conducted revealed that many patients with hypothyroidism and residual symptoms have visited five to ten physicians or more.[8]

* * *

As we have seen, hypothyroidism is a disease caused by insufficient amounts of thyroid hormones in the body. Thus, since the 1890s there has been a consensus that treatment of hypothyroidism involves restoring thyroid-hormone levels to normal. Patients should be given appropriate amounts of thyroid hormones to make up for what is missing, given their failing thyroid gland. This is well accepted by all physicians, without dispute.

Therefore, the goal of supplementation therapy is to restore the body with normal amounts of thyroid hormones and normalize its action in all organs. Achieving normal levels of thyroid hormones will eliminate signs and symptoms of the disease and will restore quality of life, without over- or undertreatment.

But how exactly is this accomplished? What do we give patients, and how much do we give?

The thyroid gland produces a mixture of iodine-containing hormones, of which T_4 and T_3 are the most relevant. Almost all thyroid secretion is T_4, and yet T_4 is not an active hormone. In other words, organs do not respond to T_4. To become active, T_4 must be transformed to T_3. T_3 is the active hormone, responsible for the effects of thyroid secretion throughout the body.

Activation of T_4 takes place outside the thyroid gland. Most organs can convert T_4 to T_3, so much so that lots of T_3 can be found in the circulation of patients treated with only T_4. Hence, the question: Which hormone should be used to treat hypothyroidism? T_4, which is slow acting and depends on activation, or T_3, which is fast acting and delivers potent effects without intervening steps?

The original treatment with thyroid extract developed in the 1890s contained both hormones. Thyroid extract is a mixture of T_4 and T_3 at an approximately 4:1 ratio. The dose of thyroid extract given was calibrated based on the resolution of symptoms—that is, the goal was to give the minimum amount of thyroid extract that eliminated all symptoms. Only after the synthetic forms of T_4 and T_3 became available could treatment be prescribed with only T_4, only T_3, or a combination of the two.

Indeed, the use of either T_4 or T_3, independently of each other, dramatically reverses signs and symptoms of overt hypothyroidism. Nonetheless, T_3 was never considered as a long-term solution for patients with hypothyroidism. The body rapidly takes in (absorbs) and disposes of (metabolizes) T_3, resulting in marked fluctuations in circulating-T_3 levels and its effects, which is not good. This contrasts with the steady circulating-T_3 levels observed throughout the day in normal individuals. Things are much smoother with T_4. Hence, it was given serious consideration since it was introduced by pharmaceutical companies.

For nearly ninety years, physicians prescribed thyroid extracts, which they knew contained a mixture of T_4 and T_3, not knowing if these hormones were closely related or why the thyroid gland bothered to produce them. After the 1970s, physicians moved from prescribing thyroid extract to prescribing T_4 as therapy. They also redefined the goal of hypothyroidism treatment, prioritizing the normalization of TSH levels over the resolution of symptoms. The T_4-to-T_3 conversion mechanism was and still is a jewel of contemporary thyroid research. All of the medical community perceived physicians who prescribed T_4 as savvy and up to date in physiology, given that they understood this newly identified mechanism of thyroid-hormone conversion.

It is indeed fascinating that the thyroid gland secretes an unfinished hormone (T_4) that must be activated (to T_3) just before it acts in different organs. This novel pathway attracted the attention of hundreds of scientists around the world. Including me.

* * *

Patients frequently ask me why the thyroid gland secretes two hormones that essentially do the same thing, and why this is important. Why not instead have just T_3, the active hormone, and keep it at stable levels in the circulation?

The answer lies in first looking at how other hormones work. The levels of most hormones in the circulation are not stable. They may fluctuate markedly in response to different cues, such as time of day, whether someone is eating or fasting, whether they are cold, dehydrated, and so on. For example, when you eat sugars, ideally your body releases insulin into the circulation, elevating its levels in the blood by about five- or sixfold. High insulin levels will in turn push sugar from the circulation into different organs until it returns to normal.

Nothing like that happens with thyroid hormones. The T_3 levels in circulation are relatively stable throughout the day and night, under most conditions. However, if T_3 levels are stable, how can T_3 modify the different bodily functions that are sensitive to it? This is a question that bothered thyroid scientists for a long time, but the issue was resolved with a better understanding of the mechanisms that explain T_4-to-T_3 conversion.

Several years ago, P. Reed Larsen (I will introduce him more fully later) and I prepared an editorial that addressed these points, "Tranquil Plasma Surrounding an Intracellular Storm."[9] This was meant to highlight how the relative stability in T_3 levels in the circulation contrasts with a stormy environment inside some organs, which more resembles a fast roller coaster. Yes, not all, but *some* organs can accelerate the local conversion of T_4 to T_3 and hold on to the T_3 for several hours without affecting T_3 levels in the circulation. But when we look only at T_3 levels in the circulation, we don't see this happening. Later, my former fellows Scott Ribich and Brian Kim and I called it "an inside job," given that the real action is taking place inside those organs.[10]

For example, a postdoctoral fellow in my laboratory, João Pedro Werneck, showed that treadmill exercise accelerates the conversion of T_4 to T_3 in the mouse skeletal muscle. So that during exercise, T_4 is activated to T_3 at a faster pace. The resulting local buildup of T_3 increases the muscle's capacity to produce energy.[11] Thus, T_3 action in the skeletal muscle is customized during exercise. All of this takes place, of course, without changes in the circulating levels of T_3. Had this increase in T_3 occurred in the circulation, *all* organs in the body would be stimulated by T_3 during exercise, which would not be desirable.

In contrast, thyroid-hormone action in organs that cannot accelerate local T_4 activation is relatively stable, reflecting the steady T_3 levels in the circulation. The ability to accelerate T_4-to-T_3 conversion on demand and in an organ-specific fashion gives the system a great deal of flexibility. This would not be possible if the thyroid gland secreted only T_3.

* * *

Surprisingly, as therapy with thyroid extract was being abandoned in favor of treatment with T_4, there were no clinical trials to compare both forms of treatment. As you are probably aware, a clinical trial is a controlled clinical study to determine whether a specific drug or treatment is safe and effective in the treatment of a disease. Sometimes a clinical trial compares, head-to-head, the performance of two or more drugs or treatments for the same disease.

The available studies showed that treatment with T_4 resolves symptoms of overt hypothyroidism. However, nobody bothered to ask or test whether T_4 is superior to thyroid extract (or vice versa). Both products are older than the Food and Drug Administration (FDA) and were grandfathered in when the agency was created. Until recently, neither drug had been formally approved or regulated by the FDA, so safety and effectiveness were never formally compared.

In retrospect, it seems that physicians were a bit too fascinated by synthetic T_4 and the fact that humans can convert T_4 to T_3, as shown in 1970.[12] They quickly moved to bridge the gap between basic sciences and therapeutics without asking whether all patients were satisfied with the new treatment. We physicians were just told by our professors, in books, and by the clinical guidelines to tell the patients that they should be satisfied since their TSH levels were normal. We ignored anyone who disagreed.

*   *   *

There was one more twist to the story. After T_4 became the standard of care, physicians who continued prescribing thyroid extract were seen as old-fashioned and many times labeled as quacks. For example, I would hear from my colleagues, almost murmuring, "He still prescribes thyroid extract," or "Be aware, she treats patients with T_3," along with a funny suspicious face. It is difficult to understand how this came about. In part, it was due to the push to prescribe T_4 and the discovery of T_4-to-T_3 conversion—as in "if you don't do it, it must be because you don't understand." But it is also because, since the discovery and formulation of T_3, certain physicians have prescribed it and thyroid extract abusively. They prescribed both medications to accelerate metabolism and weight loss in what they labeled as "hypometabolic" patients who did not have hypothyroidism.

The practice of prescribing treatment with thyroid hormones for individuals who do not have hypothyroidism is ill advised, and medical societies have condemned it.[13] Unfortunately, it continues to happen to this day. The rationale for this approach is that T_3 is a very active molecule that does indeed accelerate fat burning and weight loss. However, eliciting these metabolic effects requires higher doses of thyroid hormones that invariably cause undesirable effects that can be life threatening—possibly triggering atrial fibrillation, bone loss, and muscle wasting.

I had the opportunity to witness this firsthand as an expert in a handful of lawsuits brought by patients against physicians. In the most recent one, a middle-aged woman who had never been formally diagnosed with hypothyroidism was treated for about sixteen years with doses of T_3 that reached as much as 81 micrograms per day in tandem with 550 micrograms per day of T_4 (the normal daily production is about 30 micrograms for T_3 and 90 micrograms for T_4). These doses were very large, sufficient to treat at least six patients with hypothyroidism. During all the years that the patient was treated at this clinic, her serum TSH remained undetectable (reflecting the high doses of thyroid hormones); and, most surprising, not a single measurement of T_4 or T_3 levels was ever obtained. The patient was finally admitted to the emergency room with atrial fibrillation, which fortunately was reversed spontaneously a couple of weeks later after treatment with thyroid hormones was discontinued.

Thus, physicians who traditionally used thyroid extract or combination therapy to genuinely treat hypothyroidism were hit from both sides. The practice of prescribing either thyroid extract or T_3 was confused with bona fide bad medicine and negative publicity, while T_4 was hailed as the best treatment for hypothyroidism. As a result, some physicians would admit only privately to prescribing thyroid extract or T_3 to patients with hypothyroidism.

I remember a conference on hypothyroidism in 2014, where a speaker asked the audience for a show of hands of those who prescribe combination therapy. I believe two people raised their hands in a room seated with about one hundred. During the coffee break, however, many approached me to say that they had several patients on combination therapy. Peer pressure prevented them from raising their hand. It also made a colleague of mine ask fellows and residents not to publicize to other attending physicians his practice of prescribing combination therapy to symptomatic patients with hypothyroidism.

* * *

In retrospect, it seems we took a lot for granted. T_4, at doses adjusted based on TSH levels, was introduced and became the standard of care without a clinical trial showing the percentage of patients who had their symptoms resolved. When studies were done much later, the results were disappointing. Some of the T_4-treated patients exhibited a lower quality of life and suffered from deficits in cognition, as shown in studies performed in the United Kingdom, the Netherlands, and the United States.

In addition, there have never been double-blind randomized studies assessing how T_4 ranks against thyroid extract in the treatment of hypothyroidism. The results of the first trial have only now become available and confirm that some T_4-treated patients remain symptomatic and benefit from switching to combination therapy. Back when the FDA was created, the fact that T_4 was reliable, was practical, and did not cause adverse effects was sufficient to obtain approval from the FDA. Later, it became the standard of care based on recommendations from professional societies.

It is not clear why experts did not alert physicians in general and patients that the efficacy of T_4 was incomplete when restoring quality of life and cognition. T_4 is good medicine and resolves symptoms of hypothyroidism for most patients. It is OK if it does not resolve all symptoms for all patients, *but we need to let people know that*. The FDA never asked for studies to address these critical points, despite solid evidence of patients' concerns. Only much later, around 2012, did professional societies point to the fact that T_4-treated patients might have residual symptoms, while nonetheless reaffirming T_4 as the standard of care.

I was practicing medicine in the 1980s; honestly, the effectiveness of T_4 was dogma and never questioned by anyone. I learned this from my professors and simply applied it in practice. Little did I know, T_4 *had not* been thoroughly examined by the FDA at that time. In my mind—and I assume my colleagues' as well—knowing that T_4 is converted to T_3 made it an obvious first choice and justified the leap. Again, the discovery of the mechanisms governing T_4-to-T_3 conversion, and how this is critical to regulating TSH secretion, caused such an impact on the field that we believed ourselves physiologically knowledgeable and—consequently—became less responsive to patients' complaints.

I remember how these novel mechanisms and the role they played in TSH regulation mesmerized me; they mesmerized my colleagues as well. At the same time, I also remember colleagues rolling their eyes at the thought that T_4-treated patients could experience residual symptoms. I am embarrassed to admit, but I did this too.

*　*　*

This crisis—namely, the residual symptoms of millions of hypothyroid patients who are considered optimally treated by their doctors—developed after changes in the treatment for hypothyroidism were introduced. In the next chapter, I explain how pharmaceutical companies accelerated this change and influenced physicians to build T_4 brand names that were repeatedly sold for huge profits.

CHAPTER 2

Pharmaceutical Companies and Their Influence

T_4 was identified at the beginning of the twentieth century, and in the late 1950s, Flint Laboratories, a subsidiary of Baxter Travenol Laboratories, introduced a new brand of synthetic T_4, Synthroid, to the American market, which had seen other brands of T_4 since 1927.[1]

In the 1950s, the FDA approval of new drugs was not as rigorous as it is today. It was a simplified process, and Synthroid was approved without formal clinical trials that compared its effectiveness or superiority to the alternative treatment, thyroid extract.

In 1962, the bar for safety testing was moved up, and proof of efficacy was required for the first time. But the law applied only to new drugs. Again, Synthroid was grandfathered in, and manufacturers were never asked to submit trial data or go through the official FDA approval process.[2]

After Synthroid was introduced, physicians only seldom prescribed it or other T_4 brands. Around that time, physicians had a hard time managing patients on T_4, as the relationship between T_4 and T_3 wasn't clear. They understood well and had been using thyroid extract for decades to successfully treat hypothyroidism, albeit plagued by inconsistencies and lack of potency standardization.

The 1970 discovery that T_4 is transformed to T_3 in many organs, and that patients treated with only T_4 build up substantial levels of T_3 in the circulation, changed the treatment of hypothyroidism.[3] This discovery clarified the relationship between T_4 and T_3 and triggered widespread use of synthetic T_4. During the next ten years, synthetic T_4 would replace thyroid extract as the standard of care for hypothyroidism.

*   *   *

The speed at which the switch from thyroid extract to synthetic T_4 occurred has become a prime example of an extremely successful marketing campaign, one launched by Flint to build and maintain the Synthroid brand name. The campaign has become the subject of a case study developed at Northwestern University's Kellogg School of Management.[4]

Pharmaceutical companies have known for years that the way physicians treat patients can be influenced by educational activities such as lectures and publications. These companies have deep pockets and ready access to unlimited resources. Thus, it has been common industry practice to use sophisticated methods to persuade physicians to prescribe their products. In the 1970s, pharmaceutical companies had much more freedom to operate; they could be aggressive. (This has changed over time, due to greater regulatory restrictions put in place by physicians' societies and academic medical centers.) Flint, with Synthroid, was no different. They lobbied physicians, key opinion leaders, and professional associations in the thyroid field.

The campaign was based on building influential relationships with an extended network of physicians and patients. Like with any other pharmaceutical company, Synthroid representatives were allowed in physician offices and academic medical centers for in-person meetings with physicians, frequently distributing free samples and generous perks such as dinners and travels.

The goal was to transmit the message that Synthroid was a superior synthetic molecule that could be accurately delivered to restore thyroid-hormone levels in patients with hypothyroidism. Forget about the old pig's thyroid extract. The company offered color-coded tablets with multiple doses, simplifying the process of dose adjustment. Thanks to another timely scientific breakthrough, the doses of T_4 were now calibrated to normalize TSH levels in the circulation. Altogether, treatment of hypothyroidism shifted fast, from grains of thyroid extract to micrograms of synthetic T_4.

It was all about influencing physicians' prescribing behavior. Pharma representatives and a handful of selected expert physicians carried Flint's carefully formulated message of Synthroid's superiority to all healthcare providers in the country. The problem is, there were no clinical studies to back up the message. Synthroid had not been formally tested against thyroid extract for efficacy or safety.

* * *

Flint had an army of pharma representatives that covered the United States, reporting to a few district managers and the central office. In the summer of 2021, I spoke at length to a person I will call Jon, one of the key individuals involved in this network. The pharma representatives reported to Flint's corporate marketing/ sales arm. Their job was to schmooze with physicians, fostering professional and social relationships with physicians. While visiting physicians' offices, they waved the 1970 study showing T_4-to-T_3 conversion in humans and explicitly said that prescribing T_4 normalizes all parameters of thyroid function, including TSH, T_4, and T_3 levels in the blood.[5]

Pharma representatives stressed that thyroid extract came from cows and pigs and that the potency of the tablets depended on the season during which the thyroids had been harvested. "You want your patient to be on something synthetic, predictable, proven to provide adequate amounts of both thyroid hormones," was the sentence rehearsed at the main office.

Jon told me that they routinely used other physicians to reinforce their message. The "academics" were physicians known as key opinion leaders, or "thought leaders," in the thyroid field. These were respected physicians with national stature, as well as local "high-prescriber" physicians within certain communities— who all could influence other physicians through their professional status and high-volume practices. The district managers always had a list of fifteen to twenty opinion leaders to work with, known as the speakers' bureau. Everyone on the list had agreed to participate in marketing events. District managers and pharma representatives would drive or fly these physicians to luncheons, dinners, or other social events involving doctors in hospitals or communities.

During these events, the opinion leaders would use a "slide kit"—prepared by Flint's marketing/sales, reviewed by their medical department and approved by legal—to speak about the treatment of hypothyroidism and the advantages of T_4 over thyroid extract and, in the end, collect an honorarium (paycheck). That is why pharma representatives and legal would go berserk every time physicians refused to use the slide kit or wanted to mix some of their own slides into the deck, a second source familiar with the process told me.

Because of their status in the field, their message was very influential. The other physicians and the pharma representatives were amazed at how smart these leaders were. After all, these were hand-picked, high-caliber physicians, all members of prestigious professional endocrine and thyroid societies. Jon remembers those times as an era in which there was a very tight relationship between industry and academia, a friendship, "with an understanding of what Synthroid owners needed to have said—and I never saw it not said."

These events were so critical to Flint's marketing strategy that the performance of the pharma representatives and their district managers was assessed through the number of events they organized per month, the number of physicians per event, and, of course, by the gross sales in the areas under their responsibility. Jon recalls that sometime in 1981 they celebrated the first month ever in which sales topped $1 million.

*   *   *

The influence over the physicians did not stop with the speakers' bureau. It extended well into professional societies, their meetings and conferences, and their research. The American Association of Clinical Endocrinology, the American Thyroid Association, the Endocrine Society, the Hormone Foundation, the Thyroid Foundation of America, and the Thyroid Cancer Survivors' Association, one way or another, received funds from Synthroid's manufacturer.[6]

Professional medical associations run on a low budget that supports office staff, research, and educational initiatives, such as conferences, symposia, guidelines, research grants, and other scholarly programs. The sources of income are few and well known: membership dues; donations from members, directed or not to specific endowments; royalties from journals owned by the society; and *support from pharmaceutical companies.*

It is quite expensive to bring a thousand physicians together in a luxury hotel or large convention center every year. Physicians pay for registration fees and their own travel expenses, but those alone don't cover all the expenses involved. Here is where the pharmaceutical companies do leverage influence. In those days, they were allowed to fly speakers and pay for the organization of specific symposia during the event—something that rarely happens these days. Professional societies expanded tremendously during those years.

*   *   *

To influence the professional medical associations, Flint formulated a very different strategy, deployed through the corporate medical arm, independent of the marketing/sales arm. This was smart, and a lot of good was done with the support provided by the makers of Synthroid. They had a chief academic liaison whose job was "to give money away with common sense and no strings attached"—in other words, "nonpromotional." This is how a person very familiar with the program described it to me. The jewel of it all was a company-sponsored but independent organization, the Thyroid Research Advisory Council, or TRAC, which was devoted to supporting North American physician-scientists and clinician-scientists in the thyroid field.

TRAC ran from 1988 through 2002 and distributed $10 million in research support. It is largely unknown to the thyroid community today, but it had a major impact on thyroid research at the time. TRAC accepted research proposals regularly, which were reviewed and ranked by the eight TRAC members—thyroid investigators and a Flint scientist. The TRAC members had impeccable credentials and were among the most influential thyroid scientists in the country. Throughout its life, the council met thirty-three times and reviewed 383 proposals, of which 98 were funded for one or two years at an average of $70,000 per project. These numbers are huge, second only to the extramural NIH support. Discoveries that directly benefited patients with hypothyroidism were made thanks to the TRAC program—eighty-six scientific publications in peer-reviewed journals overall. Scientists used TRAC resources to generate preliminary data and later submit larger proposals to the NIH. Looking at the list of recipients of TRAC support, I see almost all of today's thyroid leaders. This was a brilliant example of a successful partnership between the pharmaceutical industry and the medical community.

The "Fellows Conference" was another successful initiative that transformed the thyroid field. The American Thyroid Association traditionally invites to their annual meeting dozens of endocrinology fellows (physicians who are in training to be endocrinologists) from around the country, to attend a full-day training program and the annual thyroid conference. The association paid for travel and housing expenses, making this program highly competitive. The makers of Synthroid approached the association and offered to pay for an enhanced program to the tune of $350,000 to $400,000 per year!

There were other things. Through the Endocrine Society, Flint (and later Boots) awarded a $50,000 research grant every year to the best presentation by a young physician during their annual meeting. They would also pay travel expenses to speakers—chosen by the Endocrine chiefs (not by the marketing department)—to visit different endocrine services around the country and give educational lectures to doctors and physicians in training. There were no strings attached. As a former chief of two endocrine services, I utilized this mechanism several times.

*　*　*

The multipronged approach initiated by Flint, through its corporate marketing, sales, and medical arms, had immediate and long-lasting effects. T_4 replaced thyroid extract and was adopted as the standard of care by every professional association in the thyroid and endocrine fields, even though superiority trials were never performed. T_4 was featured as the only option to treat hypothyroidism in clinical guidelines prepared by professional medical societies. Its prestige remains today. The United States'

T_4 market has capped at about \$5.9 billion in 2020 retail dollars. The American market has been the largest, and most likely will not change even as the other parts of the world use more T_4 and begin to see some price increases.[7]

* * *

Jon's routine during those days also included visiting physicians' offices around his district. Thousands of them. In the offices, while he waited for a physician to see him, he dropped off free samples and promotional pamphlets, and also talked to patients in the waiting area. At some point, he became puzzled by what he heard from patients—things such as "my brain does not seem to work as sharp as it used to" or "the doctor is having difficulty stabilizing me on a strength." Jon thought to himself that something was wrong with this picture. Doctors questioned if the patients were taking the medication every day; patients would swear that they were.

This all surprised Jon. He believed T_4 was the right treatment for hypothyroidism and had never heard from the key opinion leaders that patients could experience residual symptoms. To get clarification, he tactfully asked some physicians who were closer to him about what was going on. He figured they were certainly hearing similar things from the patients. They were. But they were dismissive, saying that TSH levels were normal.

At the same time, one of those physicians told Jon that some patients still required T_3. Jon was surprised by this too. He then spoke to patients who were receiving thyroid extract, and they seemed not to have the same problems that the T_4 patients were having. Jon told me he thought, "It does not take a rocket scientist to figure that one out." But the Synthroid marketing strategy with the opinion leaders was strong; it was gospel.

* * *

Ten years later, in the early 1980s, having won the battle over thyroid extract, the next major problem for the Synthroid brand was looming competition from less-expensive brands and generics. Synthroid's patent had expired years earlier, but its approximate 85% share of the American market was protected by something stronger than a patent: the bioequivalence barrier.[8] I will explain.

The FDA considers generics equal to and interchangeable with the name brand. This is known as bioequivalence, and started in 1984 with the Hatch–Waxman Amendments. Once the FDA adds a new product to their list of bioequivalence, states may then allow pharmacists to exchange products on that list. For example, when a physician prescribes Synthroid to a patient, the pharmacist can fill in the prescription with a generic or another bioequivalent brand, which is typically much cheaper. Doctors could still stop this if they wanted to, by simply writing "no substitution" on the prescription; but, as a rule, the application of the Hatch–Waxman Amendments has saved billions of dollars to consumers.

In 1986, the British company Boots Pharmaceuticals was in negotiations to purchase the Flint Laboratories unit from Baxter for a whopping $555 million.[9] While Boots and Flint were negotiating a deal, Daniels Pharmaceutical in Florida was seriously working on a new brand name of T_4. They were known for making a veterinary T_4 called Soloxine but ventured into the human market with a new product named Levoxyl, which was accepted by the FDA as being bioequivalent to Synthroid.[10] Their next move was to ask New Jersey to allow substitutions by pharmacists within the state.

Jon told me that, at that moment, Flint panicked. They feared that approval by New Jersey would open the door to other states to do the same, which could put the whole deal with Boots in jeopardy. Jon said that "Stop Levoxyl" became the directive. They sent their managers and even a high-caliber thyroid expert to meet with New Jersey representatives to advocate for Synthroid—for no bioequivalence to be issued.

In the end, the Flint–Boots deal went through but New Jersey approved Daniels's submission. Daniels knew by then they had a product for human patients that could put a dent in Synthroid's market. One by one, the states approved Levoxyl into their formularies. In turn, Boots, the new owner of Synthroid, knew by then they had a problem.

Once approved, the strategy for Levoxyl was simple: just let physicians know that there was an FDA-bioequivalent T_4 alternative to Synthroid at one-third the price! According to Jon, Daniels never paid a physician to speak on behalf of Levoxyl, but he told me they did support professional associations—they gave the first $10,000 to help create the American Association of Clinical Endocrinology, which started in Florida, also the home state for Daniels Pharmaceutical.

Boots wanted to stop the advance of Levoxyl and generic formulations of levothyroxine into Synthroid's market. How could they do it? Their first approach was marketing. They used the mechanisms they inherited from Flint to influence physicians and patients alike and launched a strong offensive against other T_4 brands and generics. They claimed that Synthroid was superior and other preparations were not, in fact, bioequivalent. But there would be more. Much more.

* * *

I was practicing around this time. The multipronged approach launched by Boots was working. Roadblocks to prescribing anything other than Synthroid came from everywhere. I have always prescribed generic T_4 to my patients. But many patients resisted, thinking I wanted to give them something cheap, less effective. In many cases, they had been told by other doctors or had read in the media that Synthroid was superior to the generic formulation. I also heard this from many of my colleagues; hence, superiority justified its relatively higher price. After all, the strategy had worked against their historical primary competitor, the thyroid extract.

However, thyroid extract did have its share of problems (such as variability of potency). But Boots did not have much on the T_4 generics or Levoxyl to work against. The message of consistency and accuracy originally crafted by Flint was good, but they needed more. They needed data to convince regulatory agencies and physicians.

Hence, in 1988 the corporate marketing/sales arm of Boots commissioned a study from two scholars from the University of California, San Francisco (USCF): Betty J. Dong, a pharmacy professor, and Francis Greenspan, a renowned endocrinologist and thyroid expert in the Department of Medicine. The study was to compare the bioequivalence of Synthroid, Levoxyl, and two T_4 generics in twenty-two women with hypothyroidism during six months. Boots paid for the study, but there was a catch—Dong was asked to sign a nondisclosure agreement where she agreed not to publish the findings without Boots's explicit permission. "She shouldn't have signed the clause and did so naively. She had consulted colleagues, but not a lawyer," the *Wall Street Journal* later reported she had admitted.[11]

It took an unusually long time for anyone in the public to hear about the results of the study. Then, in April 1996, we learned through the reporting of Ralph T. King, a staff reporter of the *Wall Street Journal*, that the study had been completed years earlier but its publication had been blocked by Boots. They wouldn't give Dong permission to publish. The results were "not good," and the timing was "just not right." At stake was the six-hundred-million-dollar US market, and an impending sale of Synthroid to Germany's BASF for the lofty price of $1.4 billion.

Ralph King reported that the Dong study revealed that Synthroid and three other drugs were bioequivalent, essentially interchangeable. Furthermore, the study design, results, and interpretation had gone through extensive review by USCF experts not connected with it, and that it had been cleared for publication.

Dong and her team did what anybody else in her place would have done. They prepared a manuscript with the results and submitted it for publication in the prestigious *Journal of the American Medical Association* (*JAMA*). *JAMA* had at least five different peer reviewers vet Dong's manuscript. It was accepted and scheduled for publication in the January 25, 1995, issue. The authors were happy—they had the page proofs to show off.

But the paper was not published. Boots exercised their contractual right to stop publication and aggressively campaigned to discredit it and suppress its conclusions. Boots claimed the study's conclusions were to be dismissed because of missteps in patient management and data analysis. "I did what I had to do," the Boots executive who launched the study is quoted as saying in the *Wall Street Journal* article. "I stopped a flawed study that would have put millions of patients at risk."

The deal with BASF went through in March 1995, and its former drug division became part of the Knoll Pharmaceutical Company, a BASF unit in Mount Olive, New Jersey. Boots said the research was disclosed and discussed in the sale negotiations. Ralph King, in his report to the *Wall Street Journal*, said that Boots executives declined to speculate on how the publication of the Dong study might have affected the sale to BASF. But an analyst interviewed for the article said publication would have been a "disaster" for Boots. "It could have substantially lowered the valuation of the transaction and accelerated the decline of the brand," he said.

* * *

Throughout the study, there was contention between Boots executives and the team of UCSF investigators. Early on, in 1989, while the volunteers were being recruited, Massachusetts was considering adding Levoxyl to its formulary, just as New Jersey had done a few months earlier. Boots asked Dong for preliminary data from her study, hoping to dissuade Massachusetts officials. Dong said no. Disclosing data before the clinical trial was completed would compromise the blinding safeguards of the trial used to prevent bias. Indeed, this is justified only if patients are endangered.[12]

In late 1990, after the study was completed, Dong turned the data over to Boots and they learned that the four T_4 products were bioequivalent.

In response, Boots sent several letters to Dong objecting to how the study was conducted. According to the *Wall Street Journal* report, Boots eventually raised 136 technical questions. In June 1991, Boots executives wrote to Dong's division head, saying that the study should be terminated. Next, they hired two consultants, who concluded the execution of the study was seriously flawed, citing questionable practices by the investigators.

This triggered UCSF to launch its own investigation. About a year later, around 1992, Scott Fields, an investigational drug pharmacist and a member of the UCSF committee overseeing clinical trials, called most discrepancies "minor and easily correctable," the *Wall Street Journal* report said.

In January 1994, Dong had incorporated all the comments and criticisms she received from Boots and sent a final draft of her manuscript for their analysis. Their executive team circled the wagons and went into damage-control mode. The company's vice president of marketing fired off several letters, calling his team into action. A letter was sent to Dong asking of any conflicts of interest she might have. Not satisfied, Boots hired investigators to find out any support provided to Dong, her division, and the

UCSF School of Pharmacy. Boots believed the UCSF team had leaked information to the maker of Levoxyl, but the investigation was "inconclusive."

Then Boots proposed changes in the manuscript. But, the *Wall Street Journal* reports, both Greenspan and Dong rejected the proposal. As a last resort, Boots threatened the authors with a lawsuit based on the nondisclosure clause in the contract, but the university lawyers were standing by the authors.

In the first week of 1995, the night before the article was to go to the printer, Dong got a call from an aide to UCSF's newly appointed attorney to handle the Boots matter. She was urged to comply with the nondisclosure—essentially reversing the stand taken by the previous attorney. Failure to comply, the aide warned, could lead Dong and the article's six coauthors to defend themselves in court, with no help from the university. Faced with the prospect of a lengthy legal dispute with a billion-dollar company, the authors gave in. Dong wrote a letter and telephoned *JAMA* instructing its editors to pull the plug on her article.

Great frustration overcame the team of investigators at UCSF. They could not publish the study they worked on for years; friends were calling about rumors and the firms' inquiries. But nothing prepared them for seeing their study published by Boots employees in a sixteen-page article, without acknowledging the people who performed the study. Worse, it was published as a reanalysis of the data generated by the UCSF team, but reaching the opposite conclusion—that that the preparations were "therapeutically inequivalent."[13]

Then, two years later, another surprise: under pressure by the FDA—who at this time knew that Knoll had an alternative analysis of the Dong study, which the company had not disclosed—the new executive team at Knoll negotiated with UCSF's chancellor and agreed not to further block the publication of the clinical trial in *JAMA*, as reported by Lawrence K. Altman in the *New*

York Times. *JAMA* published the study without any changes in the proof that was set two years earlier. The study confirmed that for most patients the less costly generic forms of the drug worked just as well as Synthroid and another brand name, Levoxyl, which is similar in price to the generic drugs. Dong and her colleagues said that, based on their results, more than $350 million could be saved each year if doctors prescribed generic forms of T_4 for most patients.[14]

* * *

The Dong publication was accompanied by an editorial and several letters and respective responses. The editorial, titled "Thyroid Storm," confirmed that Boots had waged a campaign to discredit the work, refusing permission to publish the findings.[15] The editorial, signed by Drummond Rennie—a nephrologist, the deputy editor of *JAMA*, and an adjunct professor of medicine at UCSF—scolded the university for not defending the researchers and academic freedom in the dispute. The university should have "immediately and staunchly defended" academic freedom and backed its faculty on such a basic issue, "notwithstanding the language of the contract," the journal's editorial said.

The FDA also came under attack in the editorial, for its hands-off approach regarding thyroid drugs. Setting T_4-specific standards of drug bioavailability, for example, would help physicians determine whether generic forms work as well as brand names.

Real-world experience shows that brand names and generics are equally capable of treating hypothyroidism. But they may not be bioequivalent for all patients. The T_4 molecule is identical among all preparations, but the way the tablet is prepared and its contents (filler) are different. Thus, in theory, the amount of T_4 coming into your body every day can be slightly different depending on the T_4 product.

For an uncomplicated patient (someone who is not reporting residual symptoms), minor swings in TSH levels (within the normal reference range) from time to time are acceptable. This is what the Dong study implied. But it would not be acceptable for sensitive patients. For example, I've had patients for whom an adjustment of half a tablet per week made a difference. Thus, it is an established consensus that patients should, as much as possible, stick to one product, whatever that product is, brand or generic, and avoid interchange.

A key point in the editorial was the criticism directed at the American Thyroid Association, for an excessive relationship with the drug industry. Indeed, Flint, Boots, and Knoll executives were commonly seen with the association's officers. These executives were present in strategic meetings and social events. They were intelligent and extremely pleasant to interact with. From a distance, it was hard to tell the lines separating professional and social activities. But rest assured, the pharma executives were there to do their jobs, which was to influence the physicians.

I remember around the late 1990s, during a banquet at a national meeting of the American Thyroid Association, representatives of the Synthroid manufacturers came in with a million-dollar check written to the association. The check was for research grants, and it was propped in a large frame that had to be carried by two people inside the ballroom, to everyone's applause and delight. Later that night, I saw the medical director of another pharmaceutical company that manufactured a brand of T_4, a competitor. I jokingly asked her why the Latin American Thyroid Society (for which I was the secretary-treasurer at the time), didn't receive a million-dollar check. Her response, with a smile, was along the lines of "Give me a billion-dollar market and I will write you a million-dollar check."

The *JAMA* editorial also highlighted the generous scale of research and educational grants given by Flint/Boots/Knoll to the American Thyroid Association, pointing out its inverse side: dependence. The American Thyroid Association was mentioned as receiving more than 60% of its commercial sponsorship from Knoll (a figure strongly disputed by the president of the association at the time).

But in my view, perhaps the most alarming criticism in the editorial was the fact that the journal had a hard time finding experts who did not have financial ties to the drug manufacturer to review Dong's manuscript. At face value, this indicates that Boots had an unprecedented level of control and influence over the thyroid experts—possibly a grip on those key opinion leaders who researched and educated other physicians. This, plus the financial ties to the association, painted a concerning picture.

With all fairness, I believe a healthy relationship between pharmaceutical companies and experts needs to exist. Pharmaceutical companies do not interact with patients the way doctors do. So, these companies need expert opinions. They rely on the experts to know what the patients' needs are and how best to address them.

I am a consultant to several companies that are developing or wish to develop new treatments for hypothyroidism. My job is to explain to them how the thyroid gland works, what patients need, and what the pitfalls of current treatments are. For example, I helped in the design of clinical trials—selecting what outcomes should be measured, how they will be measured, and so on. Without this type of consulting, time and money would be wasted, to the detriment of patients. This is so ingrained in the way that academic medicine works that most top-tier universities allow professors to spend 20% of their time consulting with outside companies.

However, the scenario depicted in the *JAMA* editorial seemed to be much more than this. Not being able to find experts to review the manuscript meant that Boots had cast a much wider net over a larger-than-usual group of experts and key opinion leaders through direct financial ties, including through the speakers' bureau and direct grant support to their research programs via the TRAC program.

JAMA also published a letter from the president of Knoll apologizing for having blocked the publication. He said, "We did not place equal weight on the academic implications and regret that our decision was interpreted as lack of support for academic freedom." But "flaws in the study execution and the authors' unwillingness to address them, led us to take the extraordinary step . . . of withholding permission to publish the manuscript in the spring of 1995." He also said in an interview with Lawrence Altman from the *New York Times* "that he was confident that debate among scientists about the findings would vindicate Knoll's view that the study was significantly flawed."[16] It never did. Nonetheless, two weeks later, a class-action lawsuit soon followed, with consumers claiming that by suppressing the information the company had cost them money, and for no reason. More than sixty class-action suits were settled in August 2000 for $135 million to consumers.

★   ★   ★

Boots commissioned the bioequivalence study hoping to use it to showcase their product's superiority over less-expensive competitors. But by the end of the study in 1990, the strategy had backfired, and the results were disappointing for the company. Once published, the Dong study was used by the marketing people of Levoxyl to boost their sales, just as Flint used the 1970 discovery of T_4-to-T_3 conversion to create their Synthroid brand.[17]

★   ★   ★

Trouble was just starting for Knoll. The findings of the Dong study led the FDA to look more carefully at claims made in Synthroid ads. The FDA warned Knoll that it no longer could claim that Synthroid was the gold standard for T_4 against which other brands were to be compared; claims of superiority could no longer be made.

In 1997, determined to rein in the manufacturers of thyroid drugs, the FDA ordered companies making thyroid drugs to get approval for them as "new drugs." Companies had three years to put together an application for approval. But again, *no clinical trials were required.* Instead, the companies would only have to demonstrate product consistency, with a shelf life of at least six months. This was in response to complaints filed by patients that their doctors were having a difficult time adjusting their dose— patients were getting either too much or not enough of their T_4 medication. Jon, the Flint employee involved in Synthroid operations, had heard this firsthand from the patients he met while waiting to speak to physicians.

*   *   *

The manufacturers for Levothroid, Levoxyl, and Unithroid—all less-expensive brands of T_4—submitted quality data and received approval from the FDA in August 2000. However, the manufacturers of Synthroid refused to file a new-drug application. They appealed and received a one-year extension of the original three-year deadline, now pushed to August 2001.

While this was happening, BASF Pharmaceuticals was trying to sell Synthroid to Abbott Laboratories. And in March 2001, BASF's pharmaceutical operations, which included Knoll Pharmaceuticals, were sold to Abbott for $7.2 billion. Just one month later, Abbott learned that the FDA denied the appeal, raising the real possibility that Synthroid could be taken off the market. In June 2001, the *Wall Street Journal* and the *New York Times* published articles questioning the future of the blockbuster drug.[18]

Once again, the endocrine and thyroid professional societies came to help. The societies with which Synthroid manufacturers had built a network of influence expressed concerns that patients would be placed at risk if Synthroid was taken off the market, despite the availability of other brand names and generics. The president of the American Association of Clinical Endocrinology wrote a letter to the *Wall Street Journal* ensuring that Synthroid was both safe and reliable. The FDA backtracked and gave Abbott another two-year extension. Abbott then filed the new-drug application, and Synthroid received formal FDA approval in July 2002.[19]

* * *

The tides had turned. Up until the late 2000s, few mechanisms regulated the relationship between healthcare providers and pharmaceutical companies. This has changed since January 2009, when new Pharmaceutical Research and Manufacturers of America (PhRMA) ethics guidelines were introduced. For at least fifteen years now, access to the physicians and distribution of samples in the offices have been severely curtailed. Professional societies can still receive support from pharmaceutical companies, but in most cases, it comes as support for the organization of annual meetings and scientific programs regulated by rules prepared by the accreditation council for continued medical education.

If we look back on that period before 2009 with today's values in mind, it is difficult not to be skeptical or judgmental. However, it was a different time, and it was lawful and commonplace for pharmaceutical companies to have latitude while influencing physicians and professional societies in all medical areas. We need to keep in mind that a lot of good was done with the support that came from the pharmaceutical companies, including patient education, support to the careers of young physicians starting in the thyroid field, and direct research support—the American Thyroid Association grew and became a powerhouse, distributing millions in research support for young thyroid scientists, and continues to do so to this day (approximately $4 million during the period between 2010 and 2020[20]).

Even in this new chapter, the path navigated by professional societies as it relates to pharmaceutical companies is not an easy one. On one hand, these companies are a source of financial support for research, education, and patient care. On the other hand, professional societies do prepare clinical guidelines detailing how diseases are to be treated with the drugs manufactured by the very same pharmaceutical companies that support them. The conflict of interest, or the appearance of a conflict, is real.

The Boots–Dong imbroglio was a good wake-up call. Starting at that time, the American Thyroid Association took steps to clarify its relationship with the industry. After learning about the issues involving the Dong study, the association voted to write letters to pharmaceutical companies to request that clauses restricting publication be removed from contracts; to write to their members advising them to avoid such clauses; and to write to the FDA requesting appropriate guidelines for T_4-bioequivalence studies.

The association also took steps to make itself more independent of corporate sponsorship—an essential prerequisite for maintaining public trust. The association created a corporate liaison board, in which representatives of different sectors of the thyroid-related industry meet once a year with the board of the American Thyroid Association to discuss their relationship, hear new ideas, observe the trend of thyroid disease, and more.

In addition, financial disclosures exist for every officer and staff member of the society, as well as the members of the task force commissioned to prepare clinical guidelines. There is a guidelines committee and an ethics committee that examine every case, and individuals have been barred from voting on certain recommendations or participating in specific activities if a conflict of interest has been identified.

In the fall of 2021, I spoke to Peter Kopp, a clinician-scientist at the University of Lausanne, Switzerland, who is the current president of the American Thyroid Association. He confirmed that all those mechanisms are still in place, including the practice of disclosing at the beginning of all board meetings any new conflicts of interest.

Kopp reflected on the interdependence of professional medical societies and pharmaceutical companies and concluded that a healthy relationship must exist, with balance. Indeed, the key to this balance is to know how much a given society depends on support from the companies. The more dependent they grow, the more likely it is to become a problem. With that in mind, while I was president of the American Thyroid Association, we created the Institutional Disclosures Document, which is publicly available and details *all* sources of funds and how these funds are dispersed. In the last five years, about 15% of the American Thyroid Association's revenue came from pharmaceutical companies, of which two-thirds were strictly regulated by continued medical education rules, and one-third used to offset the costs of our annual meeting. It is up to their board now to decide what is an acceptable level of dependence from the pharmaceutical industry.

But we could do more. Today, the topics to be reviewed and the composition of the task forces that prepare clinical guidelines are selected by and do report to the board of directors. The board also approves the final product of the task force, before it can be submitted for publication. In my view, to avoid the perception of a conflict of interest, an independent group of senior members of the association could be assembled to oversee the whole process, including the selection and appropriateness of the topics, the composition of the task force, and the approval process. This would insulate the group preparing the guidelines from the group that runs the association and is responsible for its financial health and relationship with the pharmaceutical industry.

*　　*　　*

This was a look at the pharmaceutical world and the powerful forces shaping the treatment of hypothyroidism. Next, I will take you into the doctor's world, where you will learn about physicians' perspectives on the treatment of hypothyroidism. Our view can be structured in the form of clinical guidelines, which are prepared by groups of experts commissioned by professional medical associations. Yet, the associations are supported by the pharmaceutical companies that manufacture the drugs discussed in the guidelines. In the case of hypothyroidism, it is surprising to see that critical information was left out of guidelines. And two key but flawed clinical dogmas gained dominance and rapidly permeated the world of hypothyroidism during the last fifty years.

CHAPTER 3

Dogmas and Guidelines

As physicians, we learn that hypothyroidism is one of the simplest and most gratifying diseases to treat. I learned this in my first year of medical school, during a lecture on human physiology. By and large, we expect that treatment with T_4 resolves symptoms such as sleepiness, cold intolerance, constipation, and bad memory in just a few weeks. After two to three months, T_4-treated patients should be symptom-free. We have been indoctrinated by our mentors and by the medical literature that, by treating patients with T_4, we provide the thyroid hormone needed to restore bodily functions.

A daily T_4 tablet, we were told, replenishes the body with the hormones that are normally produced by the healthy thyroid gland. After a few months of therapy, patients with hypothyroidism can again enjoy the life that had been stolen by the disease. The literature and the web are full of before-and-after portraits of patients with hypothyroidism, showcasing dramatic changes caused by thyroid-hormone therapy. This T_4 dogma was established sixty to seventy years ago and remains strong to this day.

Of course, we also learned that the exact dose of T_4 varies from patient to patient, but that, in each case, its appropriate amount can be defined by the TSH levels in the blood. TSH levels inform how much T_4 is in the circulation. A minor drop in T_4 levels, as we see during hypothyroidism, is sufficient to elevate TSH in the blood. Therefore, it is commonsensical to use the TSH levels to define the appropriate dose of T_4.

In general, physicians use the patient's body weight to estimate a starting dose. Further adjustments can be made with follow-up measurements of blood TSH, at about six-week intervals. Thus, a return of blood TSH levels to normal range is an indication that enough T_4 is being supplied to the patient. At this point, the patient has reached a state of "euthyroidism" (normal thyroid-hormone status) and thus is symptom-free. Like the T_4 dogma, this TSH dogma was also established in the 1970s and has resisted change to this day.

With these two dogmas in mind, it is easy to understand why the existence of dissatisfied T_4-treated patients with normal TSH levels is unexpected. It just shouldn't be. However, we now have sufficient evidence that both dogmas must be updated. Simply put, thyroid-hormone levels are not always fully restored in T_4-treated patients with a normal TSH. And T_4-treated patients may experience poor quality of life, impaired cognition, and metabolic abnormalities.

*   *   *

In 2011, the American Thyroid Association asked me if I would cochair, with the clinician-scientist Jacquie Jonklaas at Georgetown University, the task force responsible for preparing new guidelines for the treatment of hypothyroidism. I was honored to accept the invitation. Professional societies prepare and publish clinical guidelines to authoritatively state the current best practices to diagnose, treat, and follow up with patients with specific diseases.

Guidelines consist of recommendations formulated using expert opinion and the available data from clinical trials with patients. These trials are conducted by physicians and are designed to answer specific clinical questions. For example, is treatment A safe and effective for a specific disease? Is treatment A better and/or safer than treatment B for the same disease? The recommendations contained in the guidelines are graded based on the strength or quality of the evidence available. In general, a recommendation based on expert opinion is weak. In contrast, it is strong if it is based on data from randomized clinical trials.

Clinical trials have changed medicine so dramatically that many physicians today focus only on their design and interpretation, commonly referred to as outcomes research. The goal is to formulate unbiased clinical trials that enroll sufficiently large numbers of individuals to allow for the detection of relevant differences between two or more forms of treatments. The practice of medicine based on clinical trials results is known as evidence-based medicine.

Not all clinical trials are optimally designed or have sufficient statistical power to reach unequivocal conclusions; hence the need for professional task forces to capture what is important, identify weaknesses, and then issue recommendations based on the totality of information assessed. The United States government maintains a website, ClinicalTrials.gov, where all trials must be posted. Likewise, universities and internal review boards require all clinical trials to be registered before the trials can move on with the recruitment of volunteers.

Clinical guidelines are prepared to settle controversies as much as possible and to serve as the ultimate guide for a specific disease. In general, physicians and patients look for these documents to learn the proper standard of care. But I noticed that in major academic medical centers, clinical guidelines are used mostly by residents and other physicians in training. Professors know what is in the guidelines and use them as reference mostly to teach those physicians in training. In contrast, medical care outside a major academic medical center—that is, what is available for most of the country—is provided by physicians in private practice and community hospitals. In these areas, physicians follow clinical guidelines to the letter. They are gospel. I have seen many physicians carrying a printout of the guidelines in their briefcase, or a PDF in their cell phones, ready to be pulled out during a case discussion. These documents have a tremendous impact on patient care.

While preparing for the task ahead on behalf of the American Thyroid Association, I looked for what had been done in this area. I saw that since the nineteenth century, professors and heads of services used to write books describing collections of cases in detail, explaining their way to diagnose and treat patients with specific thyroid diseases. Browsing through the major thyroid textbooks published from the 1800s to today, one can appreciate how these books evolved from a series of personal reports and clinical experiences to opinionless and content rich, with thousands of references to research and clinical studies. Throughout the twentieth century, physicians progressively shifted their focus from anecdotal observations to objective data derived from clinical trials.

I will use as a starting point the article "Guidelines for the Treatment of Myxedema" by William L. Green, a clinician-scientist at Washington University in St. Louis, given that it was published in 1968—almost at the same time that the method to measure TSH in the blood became clinically available, as well as the time of the discovery that humans convert T_4 to T_3.[1]

Green thought thyroid extract was excellent and had been used successfully for decades, but there were those well-known issues with inconsistent potency. Thus, based on his expert opinion, he concluded that prescribing synthetic T_4 or T_3 represented an unquestioned theoretical advantage over thyroid extract. Green also recognized that the normal thyroid secretion contains both T_4 and T_3, but dismissed the possibility of treating patients with hypothyroidism with combination therapy. He thought no important differences in the metabolic effects of the two compounds had been demonstrated. As far as dose adjustment, the assay to measure TSH was not yet available, and Green concluded that clinical criteria (signs and symptoms) provided a very reliable guide to therapy.

Green avoided discussing the efficacy of either treatment— thyroid extract or synthetic thyroid hormones—or their ability to resolve symptoms in all patients. It was assumed that T_4 was effective for all patients with hypothyroidism. Above all, using T_4 was practical. These views were only strengthened by the 1970 study showing that T_4 is activated to T_3, which was interpreted as meaning that treating patients with T_4 would be sufficient to replenish the body with T_3.[2] This finding set the narrative for how treatment of hypothyroidism would be approached over the next twenty-seven years.

A series of similar publications followed Green's "guidelines," largely echoing his ideas except for an important distinction on how the dose of T_4 was to be adjusted. Measuring TSH levels had become clinically available as a reference to diagnose hypothyroidism. Thus, during the following years, more and more emphasis was given to the normalization of TSH levels in the blood, and less to the patients' symptoms.

This new approach did raise some concerns. In 1976, Herbert A. Selenkow, a clinician-scientist at the Peter Bent Brigham Hospital in Boston, pointed out that TSH was really useful, but at times there were inexplicable discrepancies between thyroid-hormone levels and TSH in the blood during treatment of hypothyroidism with T_4. He stressed that TSH levels should not be used as the *only* measure of the adequacy of thyroid-hormone therapy, and that the ultimate appraisal of the optimal dosage of thyroid-hormone preparations remain a clinical judgment.[3] But his concern fell on deaf ears.

The first "official guideline" that specifically included the treatment of hypothyroidism was published in 1995.[4] The document was commissioned by the American Thyroid Association to members of its Standards of Care Committee. At that time, T_4 had been extensively used for at least twenty-five years, but there were reports, albeit anecdotal, that some patients on T_4 remained symptomatic. For example, Selwyn Taylor, a surgeon-scientist at Hammersmith Hospital in London, noted in 1970 that "a very small group of patients with hypothyroidism are not entirely well on thyroxine [T_4] alone."[5]

Based on the task force's expert opinion and relevant publications, the 1995 guidelines categorically recommended T_4 as the treatment of choice for the routine management of hypothyroidism at doses that normalize circulating levels of TSH. They also specifically did not recommend preparations containing $T_4 + T_3$, although their use was not contraindicated. So, what should an internist who is looking at the guidelines for guidance do? How should they read "not recommended" versus "not contraindicated"? This sounds like the experts were tiptoeing around the issue, missing the opportunity to clarify an important problem for the rest of us.

Although studies were available,[6] at no point was it discussed whether treatment with T_4 normalized T_3 levels or eliminated all symptoms of hypothyroidism, or whether this needed to be tested in a formal trial. In retrospect, it seems that this was the moment in which the normalization of TSH levels with T_4 officially became synonymous with eliminating symptoms, and it was done based on expert opinion, not on data.

In 2002, it was the turn of the American Association of Clinical Endocrinology to publish its guidelines for hypothyroidism.[7] By then, the work being done by Naomi Roberts, a consultant clinical psychologist at Barrow Hospital in the United Kingdom, was already published.[8] As we saw, she had identified hundreds of appropriately treated—but dissatisfied—patients with hypothyroidism.

Nonetheless, without acknowledging that T_4 does not eliminate symptoms in all patients with hypothyroidism, the guidelines noted that some patients seem to do better with a combination of T_4 + T_3; but insufficient evidence was available to know which patients with hypothyroidism, if any, would be better treated with combination therapy rather than with T_4 alone. The guidelines also stated that in general, thyroid extract, combinations of thyroid hormones, or T_3 should not be used as supplementation therapy.

The 2002 guidelines indicated categorically that patients with hypothyroidism were to be treated with "high-quality brand preparation of T_4"—a statement which I sincerely did not expect. How are we to know what is high- as opposed to low-quality brand preparation? They recommended physicians prescribe brand preparations over generics, without supporting evidence. In fact, the Dong study had been published just a few years earlier showing that Synthroid and three generics were bioequivalent in the eyes of the FDA (see chapter 2).

*   *   *

After these two guidelines were published, patients that remained symptomatic on T_4 and those who benefited from combination therapy with T_3 got confused. It seemed that task forces of two eminent medical associations had failed to highlight the fact that millions of patients unequivocally did not benefit fully from T_4 and preferred combination therapy. They thought that the existence of dissatisfied patients with hypothyroidism should have worried concerned physicians. Nonetheless, the task force remained silent. Patients were puzzled and some understandably infuriated because, among other things, many felt that an effective alternative treatment was available—combination therapy—but was being dismissed.

*   *   *

Ten years later, in 2012, new guidelines for hypothyroidism were published. This time, the American Thyroid Association and the American Association of Clinical Endocrinology jointly crafted the recommendations.[9] The document acknowledged extensive work done in Wales on hundreds of dissatisfied patients on T_4 while failing to mention that these studies were reproduced and expanded further in the Netherlands.[10] And yet, the joint task force relied on a study of *only* twenty-nine women on T_4 to state that treatment with T_4 restored quality of life to patients with hypothyroidism![11] Thus, T_4 remained the standard of care of hypothyroidism without any warnings that many patients did not enjoy a full recovery.

By the time these joint guidelines were prepared, the results of several clinical trials assessing the benefits of combination therapy were available.[12] These were acknowledged in the guidelines, and the joint task force concluded that the studies largely failed to confirm an advantage of combination therapy over T_4 alone. These 2012 guidelines were not supportive of therapy with thyroid extracts either.

*   *   *

These three official guidelines published between 1995 and 2012 did not warn physicians that a substantial number of patients with hypothyroidism on T_4 remained symptomatic. They focused instead on the fact that studies failed to demonstrate the superiority of combination therapy ($T_4 + T_3$) over T_4. It is ironic that on the flip side, not a single study showing that T_4 is superior to thyroid extract ever existed, or that T_4 restores quality of life and cognitive functions to all patients with hypothyroidism.

With the patients in mind, the guidelines could have stressed these points, could have pointed out that T_4 is not perfect for all patients. They could have been more open toward alternative treatments for those patients who remain dissatisfied. So, a warning that therapy with T_4 had limitations would have made physicians more comfortable attempting combination therapy or resuming treatment with thyroid extracts on an individual basis. Patients would have benefited from this approach.

In retrospect, I believe the acceptance of T_4 as the standard of care *without serious consideration of symptomatic patients* in these three documents was a crucial galvanizing force when it came to the organization of patients around advocacy groups. In the words of a few patients of mine, "We saw then, in black-and-white terms, that despite our suffering, serious consideration of our condition was not a priority."

*   *   *

At about the same time, the European Thyroid Association nominated a task force to review what was known about persistent symptoms of hypothyroidism in T_4-treated patients with normal TSH levels and to formulate guidelines in this area.[13] After working for two years, the task force concluded that persisting symptoms existed, and could be explained by several reasons, including the patient's burden of being aware that they were suffering from a chronic disease, and from possible associated diseases concurrent to hypothyroidism. While this sounded much like the position taken by the American societies, the Europeans did something new: they explicitly stated that residual symptoms could also be the result of the inadequacy of T_4 treatment to restore physiological T_4 and T_3 levels. Nonetheless, because there was insufficient evidence that combination therapy was better than T_4 monotherapy, they went on to recommend that therapy with T_4 remain the standard treatment of hypothyroidism.

Next, the European Thyroid Association did another remarkable thing: they explicitly stated that combination therapy could be considered as an experimental approach in T_4-treated patients who have persistent complaints, provided these patients have previously received support to deal with the chronic nature of their disease, and associated diseases have been excluded. And the association did something innovative—they explained how this should be done safely. They were careful to say that combination therapy should be instituted only by accredited internists or endocrinologists and discontinued if no improvement is experienced after three months. They suggested starting combination therapy at a T_4:T_3 dose ratio between 13:1 and 20:1, along with close patient monitoring, aiming not only to normalize TSH levels but also to normalize T_4 and T_3 levels in the circulation.

* * *

For both physicians who treat patients with hypothyroidism and patients with hypothyroidism, the year 2012 was confusing. On one side of the Atlantic, guidelines from two prominent American professional societies recommended treatment of hypothyroidism with T_4 and ignored the fact that about 10–20% of these patients remain symptomatic despite treatment. On the other side, guidelines from a prominent European professional society recognized the limitations of treatment with T_4 and offered a reasonable way out for those patients that remain symptomatic: a trial with combination therapy.

I frequently attend the annual meetings of the European Thyroid Association. Around that time, my colleagues in Europe were puzzled by the American standing. They questioned the American guidelines. It is hard not to consider a connection involving the major players in this crisis—the pharmaceutical companies, the physicians, and their guidelines. Nonetheless, science is what has led us to great discoveries in the thyroid field, and I trust that science is what will lead us out of this rabbit hole.

To understand this science, we need to start at the beginning. I will start by telling you why iodine is important and how the thyroid works to secrete T_4 and T_3. Then I introduce you to the two ways your body transforms T_4 into T_3. The next part of this book explores the essential science of the thyroid gland.

PART TWO

The Science

CHAPTER 4

How the Thyroid Gland and Its Hormones Work

It is early in the morning, and Olivia Stone, a forty-seven-year-old patient of mine with hypothyroidism, takes a tablet of 125 micrograms T_4 while still in bed. She takes it in bed because T_4 should never be taken with food or other medications; taking T_4 with meals or other meds may inhibit its absorption by as much as 50% and ultimately its efficiency. Therefore, it is recommended that it be taken either one hour before breakfast, or four or more hours after dinner to ensure absorption. She and many others take it and wait in bed.

Olivia has been taking daily T_4 tablets for the last six months now. The tablet hits her stomach and starts to dissolve. It weighs about one-tenth of a gram, and the content of T_4 is only a little tiny fraction of the tablet. The rest is filler, or excipient—substances that confer stability to the molecule of T_4—and dye to make the tablets colorful. Patients may develop intolerance to the filler or the dye, which may be resolved by switching to a colorless tablet or liquid capsule.

In a few minutes, the tablet enters Olivia's duodenum (the upper part of the small intestine), where it fully dissolves, making T_4 available for absorption into the circulation. Assuming absorption is unimpaired, most T_4 will have been absorbed in a few hours, mixing with the T_4 from tablets of previous days, already in circulation.

T_4 derived from the tablets is identical to the T_4 made by the thyroid gland. Therefore, the body handles both identically. But there is a catch: T_4 alone *is not* capable of relieving symptoms of hypothyroidism, such as cold intolerance, impaired cognition, sluggishness. Your body does not respond to T_4. After absorption, most T_4 remains in the blood and only slowly enters organs. That is when T_4 is transformed to T_3. This occurs when an iodine atom is plucked out from T_4, and it thus becomes T_3. T_3 is found mostly inside the organs, modifying the functioning of the body. That means all organs respond promptly to T_3, the hormone fully capable of relieving symptoms of hypothyroidism.

It is then obvious that the conversion of T_4 to T_3 is at the center of treatment with T_4 for all patients with hypothyroidism. In this regard, the low-tech thyroid extract (derived from pig thyroid) works slightly differently when compared to T_4, as it contains a mixture of T_4 and T_3. Therefore, patients with hypothyroidism treated with thyroid extract, or other forms of combination therapy, benefit from having some T_3 ready to act upon absorption, but must also produce T_3 via the activation of T_4.

*   *   *

Why iodine is such an important factor in our health is a fascinating story. The ocean, where the first life-forms evolved, is also the largest depot of iodine on the planet. Thus, life evolved in an environment with plenty of iodine, and even early organisms were capable of combining iodine to proteins as a way to regulate their lives. You could safely say that, after approximately 3.5 billion years, life got used to relying on the readily available iodine.

The continents are not as rich in iodine, but occasionally they are peppered with iodine from the rain. The amount of iodine that is retained by the soil depends on the soil type. This is important because the amount of iodine in the soil affects all life in that region. For example, in an area of iodine deficiency such as Cambodia, Lebanon, Madagascar, and Mali, the crops that grow and the animals that feed on anything that grows in that soil will also be iodine deficient. Thus, feeding off any type of food obtained from an iodine-deficient area will reduce your daily iodine intake and place you at risk for iodine deficiency.

As animal life expanded to the continents about four hundred million years ago, evolutionary pressure favored those organisms that could concentrate and store iodine. And that is when the thyroid gland comes into play.

Your thyroid is made up of millions of cells. Each cell is bathed by capillary blood coming from arteries, straight from the heart. This blood contains iodine absorbed from your daily meals. Thyroid cells are capable of taking up iodine and using it as a building block to make thyroid hormones. They combine iodine with a large protein—called thyroglobulin—that is made only within the thyroid gland. Iodinated thyroglobulin, as the combination is called, is stored within the thyroid gland and contains T_4 and T_3. With time, thyroglobulin is slowly broken down to release T_4, T_3, and small amounts of other poorly active molecules. Provided you ingest a minimum of 150 micrograms iodine daily, your thyroid should contain about fourteen molecules of T_4 for each molecule of T_3, which explains why T_4 is the most abundant component of thyroid secretion.

However, extensive geographical areas on the planet do not retain sufficient iodine in the soil. Sandy soils and low-clay soils contain very low levels of iodine, while clay-rich soils, organic-rich soils, and alkaline soils report much higher levels. In general, terrains that underwent glaciation have a limited capacity to retain iodine. Iodine deficiency leads to goiter, which is a compensatory thyroid growth that is meant to increase its ability to take up and concentrate iodine. For all practical purposes, a goiter is a visible lump in your neck, protruding from where the thyroid gland is located; it moves up and down every time you swallow.

Provided that iodine deficiency is not severe, thyroid growth and other adjustments in the thyroid-hormone economy sustain an almost normal life for adults in iodine-deficient areas. However, children are not capable of adapting so efficiently and remain susceptible to even mild iodine deficiency. This includes a child before birth, infants, and children of all ages. For example, as discussed, during pregnancy, there is an increased requirement of iodine, which places some women at higher risk of iodine deficiency. While this might not affect the mother directly, it will affect the normal development of the child. Severe iodine deficiency during pregnancy and/or the neonatal period leads to growth retardation and neuromotor abnormalities and can reduce a child's IQ by up to ten to fifteen points. Even mild iodine deficiency can cause a significant loss of up to five IQ points.

About two billion of us live in iodine-deficient areas. This is possible only because of iodine prophylaxis, which is the addition of iodine to our daily diet—for example, in kitchen salt. Jean-Francois Coindet, a Swiss physician in Geneva, was one of the first to recognize in 1820 a connection between iodine and thyroid. He noticed that consuming dried seaweeds or sponges, because of their high iodine content, successfully reduced goiter size.[1]

At approximately the same time, Jean-Baptiste Boussingault, a French chemist conducting geological surveys in Central America in the 1820s, noticed in the Andes that the inhabitants of the valleys of Guaca and Antigoia did not suffer from goiter, though it was common in surrounding areas.[2] He identified this exemption as being associated with the use of natural salt containing iodine. Hence, the iodine-containing salt was transported to other valleys to prevent or combat the endemic.[3]

Five years later, as Boussingault continued studying the presence of iodine in the natural salt from mines in the Andes, he recommended salt iodization to prevent and treat endemic goiter. Later, around the 1860s and 1870s, a series of successful trials in Europe demonstrated the efficacy of iodine tablets in reducing goiter in boys and girls, the largest being conducted in the commune of Albi (south of Lake Geneva in France).

David Marine, a pathologist at the Lakeside Hospital in Cleveland, Ohio, spearheaded iodine prophylaxis in the United States. Marine became interested in this subject after he noticed that dogs and farm animals in the Cleveland area had goiters. As he treated goitrous dogs with iodine, he noticed their goiters shrunk and the animals changed dramatically, becoming "active and robust," probably reflecting the transition from hypothyroidism to normal thyroid function. In the late 1910s, Marine looked at thyroid-gland sizes in a group of schoolgirls in Akron, Ohio, while their diet was fortified with iodine. He saw that giving iodine greatly reduced the size of their thyroid glands.[4] In 1924, Marine lectured on his findings, noting that the work in Akron had quickly been followed by several successful studies with schoolchildren in goitrous regions of Switzerland and Italy, dramatically reducing deaf-mutism as a result of iodine deficiency in those countries.

Sadly, it took one hundred years after Coindet's discovery for the safe prophylactic value of iodine to be established by David Marine. One of the reasons for earlier antagonism was that even a small goiter would exempt young men from military service in the French army![5]

*　*　*

When I was a medical student in São Paulo in the late 1970s, approximately one to two in every ten patients I saw at the Santa

Casa hospital had a goiter. This is because iodine deficiency was endemic in large regions of Brazil and other parts of Latin America. Since very early in the twentieth century, Latin American governments decided to use salt iodization as the strategy to eliminate iodine deficiency. This followed an 1831 recommendation by Francisco Freyre Allemão e Cysneiro that it would take a governmental effort to resolve iodine deficiency. Allemão graduated as a surgeon in Rio de Janeiro, Brazil, but decided to attend the School of Medicine of Paris, where he studied salt iodization and presented a thesis titled "Dissertation sur le goitre."

However, salt iodization requires a monumental effort that demands intense quality control around manufacturing, transport, and household storage (for example, keeping iodized salt next to a hot stove will accelerate the vaporization of iodine, rapidly reducing its iodine content). Thus, deep into the 1970s, there was still a high prevalence of goiter in Brazil.

But Brazil was not alone. Surprisingly, iodine deficiency remained a problem worldwide during the better part of the twentieth century despite government-sponsored iodine prophylaxis. In the 1990s, as a result of internal discussion within Merck KGaA (a German chemical and pharmaceutical company, unrelated to the American company also named Merck) on the persisting widespread iodine deficiency in Germany, the company initiated a public survey of children ages six to fifteen on their urinary iodine content and size of the thyroid gland. As I mentioned, a goiter is one of the earliest signs of iodine deficiency and children are the most susceptible population. Under the advisement of the Belgian clinician-scientist François Delange, the company purchased a van equipped with an ultrasound neck scanner and a freezer to store urine samples. Later, the urine was processed to measure its iodine content, which is a fairly good way of estimating iodine intake.

The original idea was to keep the van running across the country; the tremendous success of the ThyroMobil program led to its expansion, covering twelve European countries: Austria, Belgium, Czech Republic, France, Germany, Hungary, Italy, Luxemburg, the Netherlands, Poland, Romania, and the Slovak Republic. Several thousand children were studied, and pockets of iodine deficiency emerged throughout Europe. This helped tremendously in directing resources to eliminate endemic iodine deficiency.

A few years later, the Latin American Thyroid Society assisted Merck KGaA in bringing the ThyroMobil program to South America. Delange cooperated closely with Eduardo Pretell, a clinician-scientist in Lima, Peru, that had trained with John Stanbury at Mass General while planning the ambitious journey of the ThyroMobil van. The van visited 163 sites in thirteen countries, from Mexico to Argentina.

The ThyroMobil program extended well into the 2000s, visiting more European countries, as well as executing similarly ambitious programs in Africa, Indonesia, and Australia. Overall, approximately forty thousand children were studied at 432 sites within thirty-two countries. This has been an extraordinary example of successful cooperation between the pharmaceutical industry, academic leaders, and governments to the benefit of the general population.

Thanks to artificial salt iodization and other ingenious strategies—such as spraying iodine over rice fields, yearly injection of iodized oil, and guidance from public surveys such as the ThyroMobil program—severe iodine deficiency is no longer a prevalent condition on our planet. Nonetheless, mild iodine deficiency still exists in parts of Africa, Asia, and Europe, including Italy.[6] In addition, children and pregnant women are at risk for developing iodine deficiency and should be actively monitored.

* * *

The thyroid gland of a normal 150-pound individual living in an area sufficient in iodine secretes into the blood approximately 90 micrograms of T_4 and only 5 micrograms of T_3 daily. Yes, the thyroid gland secretes mostly T_4, an inactive precursor molecule, to be activated to T_3 throughout your body. But the small amounts of T_3, the active thyroid hormone, provide instant thyroid-hormone action.

After the surgical removal of the thyroid, you are no longer capable of producing thyroid hormones. Nowhere else in the body will you find cells capable of manufacturing thyroid hormones. So, immediately after such surgery, the thyroid-hormone levels in the circulation start to drop, and after one or two weeks without treatment, you will experience symptoms of hypothyroidism. By the third or fourth week, you will be severely hypothyroid.

Things happen much more slowly when the thyroid gland is destroyed by your immune system, as in Hashimoto's hypothyroidism. The near-complete destruction of the thyroid gland might take place as soon as six to twelve months, or it might take years to complete. As the cells are destroyed one by one, the daily production of T_4 and T_3 drops slowly, triggering an elevation in the blood's TSH levels. Higher TSH in the blood stimulates the remaining thyroid cells to work harder, making up for the cells that have died. When they work harder, thyroid cells tend to produce more T_3—explaining why T_4 blood levels drop faster than T_3.

That the thyroid gland secretes both T_4 and T_3 constitutes a very important piece of the puzzle in the treatment of hypothyroidism. Essentially, it tells us that to successfully mimic normal thyroid secretion, the treatment of hypothyroidism must contain both T_4 and T_3. In this sense, the utilization of thyroid extract is most similar to what the human thyroid gland does, except that the pig's thyroid gland contains slightly lower T_4/T_3 ratios (in general, four molecules of T_4 for each molecule of T_3, as opposed to 14:1 in the human thyroid).

However, the downside of thyroid extract or other forms of combination therapy that contains T_3 is that T_3 is absorbed too fast into the circulation, which, along with the slightly higher content of T_3 in the pig-thyroid extract, may cause undesirable effects. Depending on how much thyroid extract is in the tablets, the T_3 levels in the circulation may overshoot and reach levels above the reference range, possibly causing side effects such as heart racing (palpitation), fine tremor, and sweating. Doctors worry about this, especially for older individuals who might have an underlying heart condition.

Of course, this does not happen when a normal thyroid gland releases T_3 into the circulation, because it does so over twenty-four hours—not all at once. Speaking to patients who are on thyroid extract, it is clear that the undesirable side effects exist but are not common. I never had many patients on thyroid extract, but I always checked for side effects. Occasionally a patient complained, and I would automatically lower the dose and carefully readjust it based on new measurements of TSH in the blood.

Treatment of hypothyroidism with T_4 became attractive because, among other things, it avoids the peaks of T_3 in the blood. This treatment was supported by the idea that the thyroid gland produces so little T_3 that other parts of the body accelerate the conversion of T_4 to T_3 and make up for the small amounts of T_3 secreted directly from the thyroid gland. Does it really?

Well, that is an interesting concept. The deiodinases certainly can adapt to preserve thyroid-hormone action. But do they? This point has never really been addressed or discussed in clinical guidelines. And it is an important point, because T_3 is the active thyroid hormone. More on this subject later—but if indeed T_3 production is not preserved in T_4-treated patients, then the fundamental principle that underlies treatment with T_4, which has been dogma for about five decades, is flawed.

* * *

Interestingly, the thyroid gland evolved to secrete predominantly a hormone that is inactive, T_4, while preserving the possibility of secreting small amounts of T_3, the active hormone.

The bulk of T_3 production occurs in multiple locations outside the thyroid gland, about 25 micrograms per day, and it is adjustable. The thyroid's job is to produce an inactive precursor (T_4) that, at the right moment and the right place (outside the thyroid gland), can be activated to T_3. As we have seen, treadmill exercise accelerates T_3 production in the skeletal muscle of mice.[7]

The amount of T_3 that is secreted directly from the thyroid gland is relatively small, about 5 micrograms per day; but it is also adjustable. Peter Laurberg, a physician-scientist at the Aalborg University Hospital in Denmark, showed that TSH is the key element that adjusts how much T_3 is secreted by the thyroid gland. For example, the human thyroid normally secretes one to two molecules of T_3 for every fourteen molecules of T_4. Under TSH stimulation, the amount of T_3 secreted may reach three to four molecules for fourteen molecules of T_4. Thus, if T_3 production outside the thyroid gland is unacceptably low, TSH levels will increase and so will the relative secretion of T_3 directly from the thyroid gland. This mechanism is meant to preserve circulating levels of T_3, maintaining steady levels in the circulation, without bumps or valleys.

All these facts pose a challenge when the thyroid gland is removed or no longer works. The system is stiffened if you are treated with T_4 only. No active hormone is provided, and the body relies instead 100% on the mechanisms outside the thyroid gland to convert T_4 to T_3 and defend circulating-T_3 levels. In addition, based on your genes, you might have an additional impairment in the ability to transform T_4 to T_3, which complicates things even further (more on this later). This is less of an issue when patients are treated with a fixed mixture of synthetic T_4 and T_3, or with the thyroid extract.

* * *

The conversion of T_4 to T_3 can occur spontaneously. In other words, if my patient Olivia leaves a cup containing a T_4 solution on the kitchen counter near a window, she would find the next day that small amounts of the T_4 were converted to T_3, because light seems to accelerate this process.

However, the rate of spontaneous transformation of T_4 to T_3 is very slow. In the body, this reaction needs to take place at a much faster rate. Everything that happens in your body depends on enzymes, "little engines" that can accelerate reactions that otherwise would occur at a very slow pace. And, of course, the conversion of T_4 to T_3 is accelerated through the work of enzymes. In this case, this type of enzyme is known as a deiodinase (de-iodine-ase—enzyme that removes iodine). After T_4 exits the bloodstream into the organs, it is rapidly attracted by the deiodinases. A molecule of T_4 touches a deiodinase for a minuscule fraction of a second, sufficient for the deiodinase to pluck an iodine atom from the T_4. This turns it into a molecule of T_3, which is free to hang out inside the cell or to reenter the circulation.

The deiodinases are at the heart of the therapy for hypothyroidism with T_4. Two types of deiodinases can covert T_4 to T_3, and researchers studied them closely during the 1970s and 1980s: the type-1 deiodinase, or the D1, and the type-2 deiodinase, or the D2.

The discovery of D1 occurred in the 1970s. D1 converts T_4 to T_3 at remarkable rates. For about ten years, D1 was all that was known that converted T_4 to T_3. Then, in the early 1980s, a team of brilliant young investigators in Reed Larsen's laboratory at the Brigham and Women's Hospital in Boston—Michael Kaplan, Jack Leonard, Enrique Silva, and Theo Visser—discovered D2, which can convert T_4 to T_3 about a thousand times faster than D1.[8]

Together, all the D1 and D2 in your body produce about sixteen trillion molecules of T_3 per minute. Thus, it is easy to understand the relevance of the deiodinases and why their function in each organ is tightly regulated. The more D1 and/or D2 activity, the faster T_4 is activated to T_3. The D2 pathway is the main route that converts T_4 to T_3 in humans. D2 is responsible for the production of most T_3 present in your blood.

At about the same time scientists discovered D2, studies in several laboratories indicated the existence of yet another deiodination pathway, the type-3 deiodinase, or D3. This is the pathway through which some T_4 and most T_3 are inactivated, then eliminated from the body. As it turns out, there is a balance between *activating* and *deactivating* deiodinases. Whereas D1 and D2 produce T_3, D3 terminates thyroid-hormone action and gets rid of T_4 and T_3. The massive presence of D3 in the placenta largely explains the need for higher doses of T_4 in patients with hypothyroidism during pregnancy.

Despite this remarkable system of three deiodinases, work from my laboratory has shown that the thyroid alone can readjust itself and secrete sufficient amounts of T_3 to preserve its levels within normal range, even without the help of the deiodinases. In other words, D1 and D2 are not essential to maintain T_3 levels in circulation, as long as the function of the thyroid gland is normal. A healthy thyroid can do it alone.

Hence, any defects in the D2 or D1 pathway can be compensated for by adjustments in the thyroid secretion of T_3. In cases of D1 and/or D2 defects, your thyroid steps up and produces more T_3, making up for any defects in T_3 production via the deiodinases.

Besides being fascinating in and of itself, this shows unequivocally that the thyroid system is hardwired to defend and preserve the circulating levels of T_3. Given that the thyroid goes through the trouble of developing mechanisms that can dramatically accelerate T_3 production, I can only conclude that keeping normal T_3 levels must be important.

* * *

No doubt, the thyroid works to preserve circulating-T_3 levels. However, Olivia's thyroid can't adjust T_3 production. She has autoimmune hypothyroidism, which means her thyroid was destroyed by her immune system and does not function at all. (For others, hypothyroidism can be the result of the surgical removal of the gland.) Thus, while those who have a healthy thyroid can compensate for insufficient conversion of T_4 to T_3, she cannot compensate, given that her thyroid does not function. Thus she relies on the deiodinases to produce all T_3 in her body, and thus any defects in the deiodinases can be a major issue for Olivia and patients like her who take T_4. For obvious reasons, anything that impairs the D1 or the D2 pathway will disrupt T_4-to-T_3 conversion and decrease the effectiveness of T_4 to treat hypothyroidism. It most likely contributes to patients remaining symptomatic.

Throughout my career, I have received many notes from patients with hypothyroidism telling me that they have a deiodinase defect, which complicated their treatment. I am embarrassed to admit that I used to disregard these messages. First, it had never dawned on me that T_4 deiodination played such an important role in defining the response of patients with hypothyroidism to treatment with T_4. Second, no cases had ever been reported in which deiodinase defects had been scientifically documented. Now, I know better.

Today we know much more about deiodinases and their defects. Small genetic variations in the D2 pathway, such as those caused by a change in the gene that encodes D2, known as a gene polymorphism, might play a big role as well. These polymorphisms are present in a large number of individuals and compromise D2 activity significantly (more on this later).[9]

In addition, the winter of 2018 saw the discovery of the first genetic mutation in a deiodinase gene at the University of Chicago.[10] My colleague Samuel Refetoff is the world's top physician-scientist working in the genetics of thyroid diseases. Students love him, and all of us have admired him as the oracle for thyroid diseases. After describing the syndrome of resistance to thyroid hormones in the late 1960s, Refetoff built over the years a world network of physicians who regularly send him blood samples of families affected by unexplainable thyroid diseases. Refetoff and his team analyze the clinical and laboratory findings and the patient's DNA (along with the families' DNA) as if they are parts of a complex puzzle, looking for one or more genetic clues or defects that could explain the condition.

In one of our joint lab meetings, Refetoff and Alexandra Dumitrescu, a physician-scientist on his team, showed us two families who were sent to them for unrelated reasons but that they noticed had alterations in thyroid-hormone levels suggestive of a D1 problem. Sure enough, when the team sequenced the DNA of these families, they identified two unrelated mutations in the D1 gene. Next, they asked Monica Franca, one of their fellows, to recreate the mutation in the lab and test whether that mutation affected D1 activity.

Indeed, the mutation had such a dramatic effect that it cut D1 activity by half. These individuals had normal T_3 levels in the circulation, because they had a healthy thyroid gland that compensated for the impaired D1 activity. However, if any of these individuals were to become hypothyroid and were treated with T_4, their ability to produce T_3 would be reduced.

These findings are remarkable. They show that defects in D2 and D1 exist and are normally masked by the normal functioning of a healthy thyroid. Nonetheless, these defects will make life difficult for patients with hypothyroidism kept on T_4.

* * *

It is amazing how nature selected iodine to play such an important role in the lives of all vertebrate animals, including us. The idea that the thyroid gland secretes an unfinished hormone (T_4) that must be activated (transformed to T_3) before it can do anything is mindboggling. I feel privileged to have known and worked so closely with some of the individuals who unraveled the D1 and D2 stories. I use the next chapter to explain how I got involved in these studies. I explain a little bit of my career, the studies I performed, and the discoveries I made so that you can get a clear picture of what context I worked within. Because T_4-to T_3 conversion is such an important piece of the puzzle in the treatment of hypothyroidism, I also give you a greater in-depth understanding of how D2 works and how it affects TSH secretion and brain function.

CHAPTER 5

How T_4 Transforms into T_3

As a teenager growing up in São Paulo, Brazil, in between soccer games and American TV shows, my brother Salvador and I used to breed tropical fish and do simple experiments on them. At some point, we had several dozen fish tanks spread around our house. We had a small microscope for necropsies, and we read books, lots of books. That environment, and a love for biology and chemistry, are what sparked my interest in becoming a scientist.

As I mentioned, I assisted graduate students in the department of physiology mentored by Carlos Roberto Douglas as a medical student. I spent years helping with their research focused on how caloric intake and nutrients affect the thyroid. At night I pursued a degree in biology at the University of São Paulo, which gave me a much broader perspective about what I learned in my medical classes during the day.

Knowing my interest in science, my mom, Elide, saw an advertisement in the local newspaper about a scholarship being offered by the German government for medical students. I applied, and toward the end of my medical course, I spent three elective months working with Wilhelm Hasselbach, a physician-scientist director of the Max Planck Institute for Medical Research in Heidelberg, Germany. Hasselbach is best known for his discovery of the pump that moves calcium in the skeletal muscle. He was bright, kind, and modest. That is where, for the first time, I saw what life as a professional scientist is like in a rich, developed country. I was hooked.

In those few months, I learned a lot, as I studied how thyroid hormones affected the skeletal muscles of rabbits. After I obtained my MD and finished clinical training, and in many ways due to my experience at the Max Planck Institute, I decided to continue studying the fundamental aspects of the thyroid gland. I enrolled in a graduate program toward a master's in science and a PhD in human physiology at the University of São Paulo. The focus of my studies was the role deiodinases play in stress and acclimatization to cold environments. I also enjoyed seeing patients and discussing thyroid cases with Rui M. B. Maciel, a physician-scientist at Escola Paulista de Medicina in São Paulo. It was there that I met Julio Abucham, a clinician-scientist and my future roommate in Boston.

* * *

In my readings about the thyroid gland, the influential studies by P. Reed Larsen and Enrique Silva, the two physician-scientists at the Brigham and Women's Hospital, impressed me a great deal. Larsen was a renowned Howard Hughes Medical Institute investigator, and the head of the Thyroid Section, a position I would assume some twenty-five years later. Just like Carlos R. Douglas, my former mentor in Brazil, Silva was a Chilean expat; he had come to the United States in the early 1970s and worked at the Montefiore Medical Center in the Bronx under Jack Oppenheimer.

By the end of two years in New York, the situation in Chile was bad—the military dictatorship of Augusto Pinochet took control of the universities, and Silva wanted to remain in the United

States. Oppenheimer was moving to Minneapolis, but Silva did not want to move to the Midwest. In the fall of 1975, Silva attended the International Thyroid Congress in Boston, where he met Juan Abuid from Peru, one of Larsen's fellows, who spoke highly of Larsen as a mentor.

At that meeting, Silva became interested in the studies presented by Larsen. He saw that Larsen had also published a comprehensive study on iodine deficiency, which elegantly expanded and confirmed studies he had done in Chile before moving to the United States. All of this made Silva decide that Larsen could be his next mentor, and he asked Oppenheimer to contact Larsen. Oppenheimer had other plans and wanted Silva to go to work with somebody else. But knowing Silva's determination, he contacted Larsen and gave Silva excellent recommendations.

The work that Enrique Silva and Reed Larsen were to do in the following fifteen years was seismic, changing the way we understand thyroid-hormone action. They showed that the D2 pathway that converts T_4 to T_3 not only affects T_3 levels in the circulation but also controls how much T_3 is inside different organs. They discovered that in the brain, for example, there is so much D2 that the levels of T_3 are higher than in other organs.[1] Their work was innovative, a real paradigm shift. As with any change in perspective, there was resistance. They both told me that a reviewer of their first publication on this subject was so skeptical, the person wrote that continuing with this line of work could jeopardize their careers.

Their studies in rats showed that in some parts of the body, D2 deiodinases produce so much T_3 that substantial amounts of T_3 remain inside the organ—where it was produced—for more than twelve hours. In these cases, because T_3 stays localized for an extended period, T_3 can act in the same organ where it was produced before it ever enters the circulation. Their work revealed that organs that express D2 have enhanced thyroid-hormone action, as these organs contain T$_3$ that has entered from the circulation mixed with T$_3$ produced locally.[2]

Larsen and Silva immediately understood this property of D2 as being instrumental in two ways, based on two organs:

- (1) In the pituitary gland, where TSH is produced. There, the presence of D2 makes it possible for the secretion of TSH to be regulated by T$_4$ in circulation. T$_4$ is taken up by the pituitary gland and converted to T$_3$ via D2 so that the levels of T$_3$ inside the pituitary gland reflect the levels of T$_4$ in the circulation. Thus, a drop in circulating-T$_4$ levels reduces T$_3$ levels inside the pituitary gland, triggering an increase in TSH secretion.

- (2) In the brain, a tissue that is exquisitely sensitive to thyroid hormones. There, the presence of D2 increases the local amount of T$_3$, ensuring that sufficient levels of T$_3$ are present all the time. In addition—and perhaps more important—D2 activity is adjustable. It accelerates when circulating-T$_4$ levels drop. A faster D2 pathway compensates for the drop in circulating T$_4$, preserving the T$_3$ levels in the brain. Larsen and Silva interpreted this as a compensatory mechanism—again, to ensure that sufficient amounts of T$_3$ remain in the brain at all times.

However, as we think about these two powerful concepts— resulting from events in the pituitary gland and brain—we realize that they are irreconcilable. Either D2 functions to faithfully reflect the drop in T$_4$ levels (by generating *less* T$_3$), which accelerates TSH secretion, or D2 functions to minimize the drop in T$_4$ levels (by *stabilizing* T$_3$ production), which prevents changes in TSH secretion. You can't have it both ways.

Nonetheless, from a clinical perspective, it is clear that the way T$_4$ normalizes TSH is greatly influenced by the presence of D2 in the pituitary. Well, most organs don't have D2. And yet, for fifty years we physicians have used TSH (which depends on D2) as a reference for T_3 action in the whole body. It is now clear that using TSH levels to define the dose of T_4 in the treatment of hypothyroidism is far from perfect.

*　*　*

In 1984, I was attending as a graduate student an endocrine conference in Brazil, and Silva was a guest speaker. Rui Maciel pulled me aside at the hotel pool and did something I wasn't prepared for—he introduced me to Silva. (I was embarrassed for being in the pool while the conference was ongoing.) We found a table under an umbrella, sat down, and talked. Our meeting would change my life. Silva had two unpublished manuscripts with him. They were printed on heavy paper. The graphs were beautifully plotted, similar to what I had seen in his publications (later I learned that these were affectionately called "Enriquegrams" and were prepared by a professional artist). I was impressed. We also discussed some of my work, which he seemed to like. It was amazing.

After an hour of conversation, I told him I wanted to go to Boston to work with him. He said he needed to think about it and discuss it with Larsen. Silva never wrote me back; but after a few months, I called. I asked my dad if I could make an international call to the United States—a big deal at that time—and ventured to talk to the Brigham operator to find his phone number and speak to him. When I got Silva on the phone he quickly said yes, and after almost one year exchanging letters and obtaining visa documents, I arrived in Boston. It was September 30, 1985, the day after a late-season Hurricane Gloria crossed Long Island and Connecticut as a category 1 hurricane, making it the first hurricane of significant strength to hit southern New England since 1960.

*　*　*

Silva is a good man, but hard to please. His knowledge, technical experience, energy, and work ethic are also hard to beat. I sort of knew about this—Maria Jesus Obregon, a thyroid scientist in Madrid, had worked with Silva and Larsen before and gave me a heads-up. When I got to Boston, I was pleased to see that Silva was the only other person I knew who had an HP-15C (and knew how to use it), an advanced calculator for the time.

Working with Silva was very rewarding. In less than a year I had enough material for three publications. But it was also an intense time. I worked about twelve hours a day. Silva would keep his office door open to the laboratory to "monitor things" while I worked, and a few times, as I chatted with Peggy Mathews, his technician, he would come out and ask if I could talk and work at the same time. He wasn't kidding. Silva sharpened my focus and prepared me for what was to come. I certainly returned to Brazil a very different person.

A simple observation inspired my work with Silva. Small mammals such as squirrels, rats, and mice thrive in cold environments. However, if these animals are made hypothyroid, they cannot withstand the cold and die within a few hours. Small mammals defend their body temperature through the activation of brown adipose tissue. This is a specialized organ they carry on their backs that is capable of producing heat. We have this tissue too, around the main blood vessels of the neck and chest, but, relatively speaking, much less than rodents.

Thyroid hormones accelerate the metabolic rate and produce heat as well. The physician and physiologist Adolf Magnus-Levy discovered this while he worked at the City Hospital in Frankfurt am Main in 1895. Thus, I thought that the thyroid hormones could be acting in the brown adipose tissue. This hypothesis was based mostly on the recent work of Jack Leonard, who was working with Larsen at the time. They discovered that brown adipose tissue has high levels of D2, but thought it functioned as a source of T_3 for circulation, which Silva later confirmed.

Perhaps because I was in love with the role D2 played in the pituitary gland, not yet understanding its controversial aspects, I discussed with Silva as I arrived in Boston that D2 could play a role in the brown adipose tissue itself, producing T_3 locally and stimulating heat production. Silva was skeptical because a couple of years earlier, a high-profile scientist showed that thyroid hormones inhibited the function of brown adipose tissue—the opposite of what I had proposed!

I remember presenting my theory at a lab meeting. Leonard was also skeptical; he spoke loudly and made fun of me. I did not quite understand what he said, as my English was a work in progress at the time. But people laughed. Silva got mad but did not say anything. He later explained that I should have accumulated some supportive results before presenting my hypothesis. Despite this initial turbulence, somehow I convinced Silva to allow me to work on this controversial hypothesis. More important, he brilliantly mentored me on these studies, which later I presented as my PhD thesis.[3]

* * *

How D2 is capable of generating so much T_3 inside the cell, remained a mystery that was only preliminarily solved fifteen years later. Munira Baqui worked as a postdoctoral fellow in my laboratory at the Brigham and Women's Hospital. She had exceptional imaging skills and was able to prepare beautiful microscopic pictures of cultured cells expressing D1 or D2.[4] Her studies showed that D1 is located in the periphery of the cell, in the membrane that separates the cell from the outside space.

In contrast, she found D2 located deep inside the cell, touching the cell nucleus. This was unexpected. Her studies provided the first mechanistic explanation of why T_3 produced by the D2 pathway stays inside cells for many hours. This allows for a localized buildup of T$_3$ that triggers thyroid effects in those cells, accelerating the cellular metabolism before escaping to the circulation.

*   *   *

Genes contain key information as to how things in our bodies are made and function. When a gene is expressed, it instructs cells on how to make proteins, which are essential for cell function. Yes, all proteins are encoded by genes, about thirty thousand of them. Around the year 1980, there was a rush to use newly developed techniques to identify and isolate genes, a process known as cloning. Through cloning, one can package the gene and insert it in bacteria, plant, mouse, or human cells. One of the first human genes to go through this process was the gene encoding human growth hormone. This is how large amounts of growth hormone are produced and used in the treatment of children with delayed growth.

Cloning of the deiodinase genes turned out to be a gigantic deal.[5] While I was a fellow in Silva's laboratory around 1986, I remember how hard Marla Berry, a postdoctoral fellow of Reed Larsen's, worked on cloning the D2 gene. There was tension because at least two other laboratories were racing toward the same goal. She tried many strategies but after a couple of years of work had not identified the gene.

Then she switched her focus to D1, which is expressed in much larger amounts in the liver. She made significant progress, but then got stuck. She identified a DNA sequence that could be the D1 gene, but the sequence was interrupted—as if there was a stoplight in the middle of the sequence. When the cell tried to make D1 out of this sequence, it would stop prematurely and quit. Much of the summer of 1990 was devoted to solving this mystery.

After lots of frustration, Larsen shared their puzzle with Brian Seed, a scientist at Massachusetts General Hospital. Seed recalled reading that on exceptional occasions, such a premature stop means the incorporation of a rare amino acid containing selenium (a selenocysteine), and suggested Berry look into this possibility.

Without wasting any time, Berry recoded the stoplight (that is, she edited the DNA molecule) with a sequence (a codon) coding for a similar amino acid that does not contain selenium (cysteine). The premature stop was eliminated, and Berry realized she had hit the jackpot. Her work not only identified the D1 gene but also elucidated a much more important thing: how proteins containing selenium are made.[6] She published two major articles in the prestigious journal *Nature*, and years later moved to the University of Hawaii, where she became the head of the Department of Biochemistry and went on to make even more discoveries in the selenium world.

As it turned out, D1 uses selenium to attack T_4 and pluck the iodine from its molecule during the deiodination reaction. The field exploded. A few years later, Donald (Don) St. Germain, a physician-scientist at Dartmouth University in New Hampshire, cloned the type 3 deiodinase (D3) gene. He showed that D3, a deiodinase that deactivates thyroid hormones, also contains selenium.

However, things were different with D2. Leonard—then at the University of Massachusetts in Worcester—claimed that D2 was different in that it did not contain selenium. This of course was at odds with studies by Val Galton, a scientist at Dartmouth College's Geisel School of Medicine, who cloned enough of the D2 gene to show that it was a selenoprotein.

These were interesting times. The field was divided and a bit too personal, too partisan. I remember every time this issue of D2 being a selenoprotein or not was presented or debated in conferences, some sided with Leonard's work, claiming D2 did not contain selenium, while others sided with Galton's work, accepting that D2 did contain selenium. Many others were just waiting. Reviewers of manuscripts and grants were particularly nasty to the opposing views. Things were awkward, to say the least.

* * *

One day around 2001, as I was arriving at the Brigham and Women's Hospital, Larsen said that two scientists in France, Drs. Rihn and Mohr, from Institut National de Recherche et de Sécurité in Vandœuvre, had overnighted a mesothelioma cell line that contained unusually high levels of D2. Mesothelioma is an aggressive lung tumor that can be fatal in many patients. Larsen asked me if I wanted to study these cells. I said yes and gave the box to my graduate student Cynthia Curcio. We figured the cells could be used to solve the controversy, showing once and for all whether D2 contained selenium.

After a series of experiments using radioactive selenium, Curcio was able to identify radioactive D2 as a selenoprotein. We prepared a manuscript and submitted it for publication. The journal accepted the manuscript in record time, just four days.[7] The study settled the matter as to the nature of D2 protein beyond any reasonable doubt. Galton was right after all. The "prima donna" among the deiodinases, D2, was indeed very similar to the other two deiodinases, D1 and D3.

* * *

A deiodinase is a protein, and proteins can assume different shapes and formats. For example, a protein may look like a sphere, a helix, a spiral, or a sheet. If it is a large protein, then its various parts can have a different shape. Nobody had a clue at that time what the deiodinases looked like.

Perhaps because we have always focused on the differences among the deiodinases, I had it in my mind that D1, D2, and D3 were very distinct proteins. The cloning of their genes by Marla Berry, Val Galton, and Don St. German made it clear that they share some similarities, but not sufficient so that we could grasp the whole picture.

We had done experiments in the lab, but those hadn't generated much in the way of new information. My children were born around this time, and I remember spending hours working on the computer at home, keeping watch while they slept. I used what is known as an "in silico" approach—in other words, I studied D1, D2, and D3 using a computer and platforms available on the web.

One of those nights, I got lucky. I found an obscure platform that analyzed proteins based on an unorthodox method that considered the way molecules of water interact with proteins. I entered the data for each deiodinase a few times. The analysis worked every time, but the output was strange—I could not understand it.

I contacted the site administrator via email thinking that I would never hear back. Instead, in a couple of days I got an email reply saying simply, "What do you want?" A critical collaboration followed with Isabelle Callebaut, a scientist at the French National Center for Scientific Research. Callebaut and her husband, Jean-Paul Mornon, used the method they developed and predicted that all three deiodinases were strikingly similar. The deiodinases are dimers (two units), much like a pair of grapes stuck together hanging from a stem. T_4 enters the enzyme's structure, and deep inside is where the selenium is located, which converts T_4 to T_3.

In fact, the similarity among the deiodinases is so strong that

Callebaut predicted that by changing one to two amino acids located in strategic positions we could turn D2 into D1, and vice versa. Sure enough, we tested their predictions in the laboratory, and they were right on the spot every time.[8]

*   *   *

D2 is such a special enzyme, at the center of the treatment of hypothyroidism. It activates the T$_4$ that patients take daily. Above all other organs, the brain in patients with hypothyroidism depends a great deal on D2 to restore it to normal function. To illustrate the nuances in the treatment of hypothyroidism, in the next part of the book, I will take you back in time and explain when and how hypothyroidism was recognized for the first time, how it used to be diagnosed, and how its treatment evolved. I will also describe how doctors, hospitals, and governments were involved in these efforts.

PART THREE

The History

CHAPTER 6

Nature's Cures

The Victorian era was a period of industrial, political, scientific, and military change within the United Kingdom. This transformed the practice of medicine. Several discoveries had advanced medical practices, and patients seeking care had access to new diagnostic procedures and technologies. Surgery had changed dramatically, as physicians took steps to increase cleanliness and sanitation by working in gowns and masks. Doctors had started wearing white coats and stethoscopes and enjoyed the reflected glory of scientific pioneers such as Claude Bernard, known for putting forward the concept that the body has an internal environment that strives to remain constant; John Snow, a leader in the development of anesthesia and medical hygiene; Louis Pasteur, renowned for his discoveries of the principles of vaccination, microbial fermentation, and pasteurization; and Marie Curie, who conducted pioneering research in radioactivity.

As cities grew in the midst of the Industrial Revolution, there were enormous consequences for health. Death rates were high, and far worse in cities than in the countryside. Smallpox, typhus, and tuberculosis were endemic, and cholera alarmingly epidemic. Overcrowding combined with poor sanitation and often poverty left many people vulnerable to disease outbreaks.

One of the concerning endemic diseases attributed to poor

sanitation and water contamination was cretinism, an irreversible syndrome caused in young children by developmental hypothyroidism. Children with the condition exhibited intellectual disability and impaired growth, frequently associated with goiter (enlargement of the thyroid gland). Despite an impairment in their development, they would grow older and live sometimes for decades suffering from short stature and being mentally disabled.

Napoleon Bonaparte was so concerned with the large numbers of young men who were unfit for military duties due to goiter or cretinism, that in 1811 he ordered a census in one of the most affected regions in southern Switzerland. He also ordered the relocation of the population with goiter to healthier areas, distancing them from the perceived causes of the syndrome.

Today we know that this condition is due to insufficient thyroid hormones (hypothyroidism) during pregnancy and/or early childhood. It was often caused by iodine deficiency, but genetic defects can also lead to the syndrome. Thyroid hormones are critical for brain development and growth—but, at the time, this relationship with the thyroid gland was not understood.

The prominence of the condition throughout the Alps was compelling and shocking, with endemic cretinism affecting every level of society. This was captured and romanticized in Honoré de Balzac's 1833 book *The Country Doctor*, about an enlightened, rationalist doctor moved by a sense of mission to eradicate cretinism from the countryside.[1] In his 1880 book *A Tramp Abroad*, Mark Twain's character of a traveler remarks: "Well, I am satisfied, I have seen the principal features of Swiss scenery—Mont Blanc and the goiter—now for home!"[2]

In 1845, Charles Albert, king of Sardinia–Piedmont, was concerned with the problem among his subjects and decided to commission a report from a committee "to bring together all the possible information on the history and progress of cretinism."

Gallo, professor of surgery and physician-in-chief of the proto-medicat, a medical-surgical-pharmaceutical council in Piedmont (created in 1839), chaired the committee. The other members were surgeons and also mine inspectors, as well as professors of geology, mineralogy, and chemistry. They worked for six years, writing letters, gathering data, analyzing samples of water from different countries, and visiting the most affected places.

The committee published its report in 1848 and concluded that living in low-ground areas, with poor quality of air and water, caused cretinism. They recommended purifying the air by draining swamps, channeling the rivers that were prone to overflow, trimming vegetation regularly, and building houses only at a secure distance from water, which we now know are ineffective measures. They also recommended that pregnant women who had previously given birth to children with the condition should deliver in a mountain setting (far from swampy areas) and stay there for several months afterward, which again is also ineffective.[3]

But the committee did get it right by recognizing the inherited aspects of the syndrome. Their rudimentary form of genetic counseling was to avoid marriages between families with members known to have the condition. This has been abandoned with the development of neonatal diagnostic methods that identify affected children before irreparable damage to the brain has been established.

The committee members were uncertain about the relationship between goiter and intellectual disability but sensed that the environment played a role. Unfortunately, they were concerned with the wrong environmental factor, as they remained stuck on the idea that improving sanitation would prevent the condition. The concept that environmental iodine was important and that endemic iodine deficiency could lead to intellectual disability evolved much later.

Other governments organized similar commissions. The Viennese physician Joseph Škoda chaired an Austrian commission established in 1859, and a French commission was established soon after, in 1862, and chaired by the physician Pierre François Olive Rayer. The French group recorded that about 370,000 people in France over the age of twenty had a goiter and that there were approximately 120,000 individuals with related disabilities (the total population of France at that time was around thirty-six million).

It is hard to grasp the emotional, social, and economic impact that this condition had on people in those days. I tend to think that cretinism in the 1800s was viewed similarly as we currently see autism, or autism spectrum disorder (ASD). Of course they are very different diseases, but the unknown cause of the disease and the overall impact on families are relatable. ASD affects children (one in every fifty-four in the US) and is characterized by challenges with social skills, speech, and nonverbal communication, impairing the full integration of affected individuals in society. We believe that ASD is associated with a combination of genetic and environmental factors, but we do not know for sure what causes it. No treatment can cure ASD, but several interventions can reduce symptoms and improve function and independent participation in the community.

*   *   *

In England, endemic cretinism was considered an exotic disease, but there was great interest in understanding its cause. Major discoveries occurred in a thirty-to-forty-year stretch in three major London hospitals: the Royal London Hospital, Guy's Hospital, and St. Thomas' Hospital.

The Royal London Hospital[4] is an academic institution situated east in the city of London. This was the first hospital in England and Wales to be organized in connection with a college of medicine, in which medical students studied under the medical staff. The surgeon Thomas B. Curling took advantage of the opportunities offered by this unique environment to study all sorts of clinical matters, preparing meticulous descriptions of his findings. In 1850, he made significant progress toward understanding cretinism. He published the first autopsy reports of two children with a syndrome very similar to cretinism.[5] But instead of an enlarged thyroid gland (goiter), these children did not have a thyroid gland at all! He proposed that the absence of the thyroid gland was the cause of the condition. He then reasoned that cretinism could be endemic (with goiter) as observed in the Alps, or sporadic when it occurred without a goiter.

Twenty-one years later, in 1871, there was a series of cases in which sporadic cretinism (in children without a goiter) was reported in another London hospital, this time the Guy's Hospital.[6] At the time, Guy's already had an established tradition of achieving medical breakthroughs, including human-to-human blood transfusion in 1818 and the first description in 1855 of Addison's disease (an uncommon disorder that occurs when the adrenal glands, located just above the kidneys, stop functioning). The cases were reported by the medical practitioner Charles H. Fagge.[7] Like the two cases reported earlier by Curling, these cases stood in stark contrast to endemic cretinism, which occurred with large goiters.

We now know that the sporadic form of the syndrome is caused by genetic defects of the thyroid gland, impairing its normal development and/or function, and we call it congenital or neonatal hypothyroidism. This condition is diagnosed through the analysis of blood collected from the baby's foot, days after delivery. It is readily treatable with daily administration of thyroid hormones.

In contrast, the endemic form of the syndrome is caused by iodine deficiency. As we saw, iodine is needed for the production of thyroid hormones. Without iodine, the thyroid gland increases in size (in an attempt to increase uptake of iodine), but eventually gives in and cannot sustain the normal production of thyroid hormones, leading to hypothyroidism. It is readily treatable with iodine supplementation.

Fagge's findings not only confirmed Curling's ideas but also must have made an impression on Fagge's colleagues at Guy's Hospital, who now became aware that the absence of a normal thyroid gland could lead to a sporadic form of the syndrome.

One of these colleagues was William W. Gull. Gull was famous for having described another important condition, the eating disorder anorexia nervosa, and, in 1871, for having successfully treated Albert Edward, the Prince of Wales and the future King Edward VII, during a life-threatening attack of typhoid fever, which made Gull one of the physicians-in-ordinary to Queen Victoria.[8]

Just two years after Fagge's report, Gull spoke of five adult women he had seen, who had been previously healthy but "looked like" children with cretinism.[9] Similar cases were not uncommon in northern areas of England. These cases had been recognized for the first time by John Byrom Bramwell, a physician working at the North Shields and Tynemouth Dispensary, northeast of England. But not until Gull presented his cases to the Clinical Society in London was this condition definitively considered a distinct disease.

Gull published a study in 1874 in which he suggested the cause of the condition he originally described in those five women was atrophy of the thyroid gland. Inspired by the work of Claude Bernard in Paris (circa 1855) around the concept of the *milieu intérieur* (internal medium of the body) and the work of Moritz Schiff in Bern (circa 1859) about the effects of the surgical removal of the thyroid in dogs, Gull proposed that the thyroid liberated some important substance into the bloodstream.

Following Gull's presentation, a fair number of papers during the 1870s reported similar cases but a breakthrough would only come in 1877 from William M. Ord,[10] a clinician-scientist based at St. Thomas' Hospital in London.[11] Aware of Gull's description of a "cretinoid state supervening in adult life," Ord identified five more women with a similar condition. But he went one step further and arranged for an autopsy of one of these patients—the first in an adult patient with the condition. The autopsy revealed a reduced thyroid gland, about a fourth of its natural size, which indicates a malfunction. Ord also noticed that the patient's skin contained an excess of mucin (a large protein that forms gels), which gave it a jelly-like swelling. Hence he gave the condition the specific name *myxoedema* ("mucinous edema," a.k.a. myxedema).[12] Ord believed that somehow the excess of mucin caused the disease.

* * *

Physicians publicized the newly discovered disease in Europe and the United States. In the years that followed, a series of reports of similar patients were communicated not only in the United Kingdom, but also in American cities—for example, New York, Syracuse, Chicago, and Louisville—and, eventually, cities in Switzerland, where endemic cretinism and goiter were common. In the Alps, surgeons were busy developing new techniques to operate on large goiters to relieve symptoms of neck compression. But that type of surgery was feared because it was associated with a very high mortality rate—the thyroid gland is near important nerves that control the vocal cords, which if affected can obstruct airflow through the trachea. In addition, the thyroid is closely associated with four other glands that control calcium levels in the blood. Removal of these glands can quickly lead to death if not promptly treated.

Jacques-Louis Reverdin, chief surgeon at the Hôpital Cantonal de Genève and a professor at the University of Geneva, assisted by his cousin Auguste Reverdin, noticed that the surgical removal of the thyroid gland caused a new clinical condition: within weeks after the surgery, patients exhibited weakness, pallor, puffy face, and hands, and their demeanor was transformed to resemble that of an individual with cretinism. In 1882, Reverdin reported his findings to the Medical Society of Geneva. He acknowledged Gull's and Ord's findings and called the condition *myxoedème opératoire*.[13]

At about the same time, E. Theodor Kocher, the new chair of the University Clinic of Surgery in Bern, was famous for having created a new style of surgery focusing on meticulous dissection, careful control of bleeding, and strict adherence to antiseptic techniques.[14] During his tenure, he was involved in thousands of goiter operations. In his hands, mortality rates for thyroid surgery dropped from about 13% to less than 1%. For his work on the thyroid gland, Kocher receive the Nobel Prize in Physiology or Medicine in 1909. Kocher was such an authority in thyroid surgery that when in 1913 Lenin's wife, Nadezhda Konstantinovna Krupskaya, needed one (she was affected by Graves' disease), Lenin selected Kocher to perform the surgery.

Unaware of Ord's and Reverdin's findings, Kocher also noticed a similar clinical development in patients undergoing total thyroid removal, which he reported in Berlin to a congress of German surgeons in 1883. He called it "cachexia strumipriva."[15] But attending Kocher's presentation in Berlin was a London otolaryngologist working at St. Thomas' Hospital, Felix Semon. He immediately noticed the resemblance of patients with cachexia strumipriva and Ord's patients with myxedema.

Upon Semon's return to London, he spoke to Ord, and they sent a letter to Kocher with more details and a picture of a patient with myxedema. So striking was the similarity between the patients with myxedema and those with cachexia strumipriva that Kocher's assistant Otto Lanz, on seeing the photograph in the letter, thought that it was taken from one of the cases he had himself photographed in Bern! Kocher wrote back, certain that both conditions were the same: "There cannot be the slightest doubt of the analogy of myxoedema and cachexia strumipriva. I was not aware of it before, having never seen a case of the affection [myxedema]."[16]

In no time, the Clinical Society in London formed a committee in 1883 to investigate myxedema. Ord chaired the committee, which included Gull, Semon, and four other surgeons. They were tasked with analyzing discoveries and clinical cases that connected the thyroid gland to myxedema.

In May 1888, the Clinical Society met to hear the report. According to Clark Sawin, a clinician-scientist at the Boston VA hospital, in his fantastic introduction to the 1991 reprint of the report, a large crowd waited anxiously at the season's last meeting of the society. The report emphatically concluded that myxedema in adults and cretinism in children were caused by a thyroid malfunction, and that the removal or destruction of the thyroid gland could cause both syndromes. Since then, myxedema as described by Ord in 1877 has become known as hypothyroidism. If hypothyroidism occurs during pregnancy or early childhood, the syndrome may result in permanent intellectual disability (cretinism), because it occurs when the infant's brain is still developing.[17]

Hypothyroidism in adults was incapacitating, producing mental and physical sluggishness and affecting quality of life and overall well-being. In his 1894 book *Myxœdema, Cretinism and the Goitres*, Edward Blake wrote that "as a rule, whilst life lasts, it is a burden." Many patients of that era ended their days in an asylum. Physicians thought there were "undoubtedly many people confined in lunatic asylums, who [were] afflicted with myxedema, of which the mental disorder is a prominent characteristic, and who might be cured in three months by the use of [thyroid] extract."[18]

*   *   *

Before specific treatment became available, hypothyroidism frequently resulted in death—ten years being the typical length of time from diagnosis to demise. The diagnosis was not made until late in the course of the disease, when severe intellectual, neurological, and psychiatric deficiency had taken over the patient. Patients would frequently exhibit dementia, debilitating neuropathy, including speaking and hearing deficits, and hypothermia—symptoms seen only exceptionally rarely today.[19]

In the late 1800s and early 1900s, diagnosis of hypothyroidism was mostly clinical, based on signs and symptoms that are caused by low thyroid-hormone levels. While a diagnosis of overt hypothyroidism could in many cases be made just by looking at and talking to the patient for a few minutes, determining cases of minor thyroid insufficiency could be challenging, as the typical clinical features are often mild and could also be caused by other conditions. Because a solid diagnostic tool did not exist, in many cases physicians resorted to a therapeutic test, which is to treat patients for some time as if they had hypothyroidism. If the patient showed signs of improvement—and resolution of symptoms—the person was kept on the treatment for life.

Specific tests developed to assist the diagnosis of hypothyroidism were very few. To measure the metabolic rate (the rate at which your organs use oxygen) was the first and most used method up until 1960s. As we saw, the thyroid hormones accelerate the rate of metabolism; thus, hypothyroidism is associated with a slower metabolic rate—decreased oxygen consumption. Metabolic rate is measured after overnight fasting. The patient is asked to rest for a few minutes and then breathe through a tube connected to where oxygen levels are measured for the next twenty minutes or so. (I always thought this test was not practical until taking another test myself, an MRI, and then changed my mind—for the MRI, which doctors routinely order a large number, I was immobilized for almost an hour with a very loud banging noise all around.) Unfortunately, other conditions unrelated to the thyroid gland can also slow the metabolic rate, so the method was prone to give false positives and was not useful for diagnosis in all cases.

There were other, even less specific methods, such as blood count (hypothyroid patients frequently have anemia), cholesterol levels (elevated in patients with hypothyroidism), the amount of protein-bound iodine (PBI) in the blood (decreased in patients with hypothyroidism), and the relaxation of deep-tendon reflexes (the reflex triggered when doctors use their hammer during routine physical examination), which is delayed in hypothyroid patients. It seems fair to assume that during this period, many hypothyroid patients went undiagnosed and others were treated unnecessarily, not truly having hypothyroidism. Only later in the twentieth century, methods that were more thyroid specific, such as detecting circulating levels of thyroid hormones, expanded the physician's arsenal to diagnose hypothyroidism.

* * *

As with cretinism, treatment of myxedema was symptomatic, by keeping patients in a warm environment and encouraging travel to warmer places during the winter. The herb jaborandi and the drug pilocarpine, as well as tonics with iron, quinine, and hypophosphites, were also used, with some anecdotal improvement of the symptoms. However, after the Ord report and the realization that a failure of the thyroid gland causes myxedema, scientists rapidly developed a more logical and specific therapy, which was to treat patients by administering animal thyroid glands.

In the early 1890s, different strategies were tested in the treatment of overt hypothyroidism. Motivated by a successful transplant surgery in animals, Victor Horsley, a professor of surgery at University College London, advocated for the transplant of a sheep thyroid into patients with hypothyroidism. Almost at the same time, José Antonio Serrano, surgeon at the Hospital de São José[20] and the Escola Médico-Cirúrgica in Lisbon, and Antonio Maria de Bettencourt Rodrigues did just that. In the summer of 1890, they transplanted one-half of a sheep's thyroid gland under the skin of the inframammary region on each side in a thirty-six-year-old woman with hypothyroidism.

Treatment was successful, but the survival of the transplanted organ was brief; so was the striking yet very temporary improvement. The surgeons then reasoned that the beneficial effects were noticed too soon after the surgery to be credited to the functioning of the transplanted thyroid. They thought instead that the effects were caused by the absorption of the juice of the grafted thyroid gland, a remarkably important conclusion. Therefore, Serrano and Bettencourt Rodrigues proposed hypodermic injections (under the skin) of a thyroid juice to achieve the same result. A few months later, they found a patient willing to undergo such treatment. After four or five injections of the sheep's thyroid juice (extract), the patient experienced substantial improvement. They reported their findings in November 1890.[21]

Along the same lines, unaware of the studies being done in Lisbon, George R. Murray, a clinician-scientist at the Royal Victoria Infirmary at Newcastle who trained under Horsley, prepared in April 1891 a glycerin-based thyroid extract from sheep and with the help of a hypodermic needle injected daily in a woman with hypothyroidism. The therapy was successful, and its beneficial effects were soon obtained by other physicians.[22] But the method was not altogether free from objections. Hypodermic needles at the time were made of metal and were not disposable. They were cleaned of blood and reused; eventually, the tip—which was not a bevel but a cone—turned dull. Some patients shrank from the hypodermic needle, while others developed abscesses in the injection site. Additionally, physicians had to prepare the extracts themselves, though soon a commercial enterprise in Newcastle made the sterilized extracts available weekly, at a moderate cost.

After these breakthroughs, Frantz Howitz, chief physician at Frederiksberg Hospital in Denmark; Edward Long Fox, a consulting physician to the British Royal Infirmary;[23] and Hector Mackenzie, a physician at St. Thomas' Hospital,[24] independently demonstrated in 1892 that the administration by mouth of the thyroid gland served the same purpose as a hypodermic injection of thyroid extract. They were rapidly followed by others, including Edward Blake, a life associate to the Sanitary Institute, England,[25] and in the United States by James A. Jackson in Boston,[26] who reported administration of thyroid by mouth to treat hypothyroidism in 1893.

According to Murray in his 1900 book, *Diseases of the Thyroid Gland*, eating an animal's thyroid was most convenient when the patient lived in a remote place or could not afford expensive treatment. About an eighth to a quarter of a lobe from a freshly killed sheep was a suitable daily dose. It is reported that the thyroid has a disgusting taste, so attempts were made to disguise this in a sandwich or lightly fried with anchovy paste on toast or taken with currant jelly. Mackenzie gave thyroid with "a little brandy." He was critical of injecting thyroid extracts. He thought it required the most scrupulous care in its preparation. The injection sometimes produced alarming immediate symptoms, such as loss of consciousness; the prospect of lifelong treatment with these injections was sobering.[27]

Most physicians, including Murray, changed to oral administration of the thyroid gland. Murray preferred to use a thyroid extract whose potency he considered would be more stable, as he was by then preparing it from a pool of sheep thyroids. So, instead of injecting, the thyroid extract was given orally as a solution, which was officially called *liquor thyroidei*.

When the thyroid could not be administered by mouth, Edward Blake strongly recommended using it in the following way: "Twice a day, after hot sponging and vigorous toweling, the body is well rubbed all over with a mixture of thyroid extract, ether [a volatile smelly liquid used as an anesthetic], and lanoline [a wax produced by wool-bearing animals]." I am surprised the inunction worked because we now know that the skin is capable of degrading thyroid hormones at a fast pace, and only about 20% of what is applied ends up being absorbed into the general circulation. I guess they were using a lot of thyroid extract.

The efficacy of these primitive forms of treatments was profound—hypothyroidism, a previously crippling and sometimes fatal disease, could be successfully treated with thyroid preparations. However, these treatments were not practical, and they did not provide long-term relief of symptoms. They were soon replaced by daily tablets containing a desiccated extract of the thyroid gland. This might sound strange today, but the therapy that uses the extract of organs, known as organotherapy, has been used since the remote days of the famous Greek physicians Hippocrates (circa BCE 400) and Galen (circa BCE 200). During its revival in the nineteenth century, organotherapy became very popular (Harrower lists forty-two organ extracts with medicinal applications in his 1920 book *Practical Organotherapy*[28]), the thyroid extract probably being one of the most successful.[29]

Thyroid extract could be prepared from the thyroid of many types of animals and was measured in grains (1 grain = 65 milligrams), packaged into tablets to be taken daily. Hubert Richardson, a physician working at the University of Maryland, writes in his 1905 book *The Thyroid and Parathyroid Gland* that in the United States the earliest forms of thyroid extract came from cows.[30] But as early as the 1900s, the Armour meatpacking company in Chicago, with its huge meatpacking operations, ventured into pharmaceuticals and the thyroid medication arena, marketing its thyroid extract from cows and pigs (all commercial thyroid extract today comes from pig thyroids). The thyroid extract was a major success story, and it remained the standard of care for hypothyroidism during the better part of the twentieth century.

* * *

The next obvious question in the treatment of the disease was how much thyroid extract to give each patient. Adequacy of treatment was judged subjectively, based on how the patient felt. According to James H. Means at Mass General Hospital, "the object of treatment should be to rid the patient of symptoms with the smallest ration of the thyroid [extract] that will accomplish this purpose."[31] This strategy, however, invariably led to overtreatment. Richardson recommended starting with 1-grain doses three times a day to a final dose of 9 grains a day, which today would be sufficient to treat at least four adult patients with hypothyroidism.[32]

Physicians were aware of frequent "untoward symptoms," nervousness, precordial pain, and/or palpitation, an indication that the dose of thyroid extract had to be reduced. From the beginning, they realized that they had to be extremely careful with dosing thyroid extract, as the line separating effective treatment from overtreatment was a thin one. Since the early days of this treatment, physicians prescribed the extract in gradually increasing amounts, up until clinical evidence of thyrotoxicosis had developed (headache, palpitation, anxiety, and angina). Therapy was then withdrawn and resumed later at a lower dose. Some physicians would automatically prescribe monthly one-week extract holidays; others would fractionate the doses of extract, to be given two or three times a day.

Many hypothyroid patients could not tolerate starting with a full dose of thyroid extract. For patients with severe hypothyroidism, physicians would first stabilize any preexisting heart conditions, even including a short period of bed rest before starting with the extract. With time, physicians more and more used laboratory tests to guide the supplementation dose, minimizing the problem of overtreatment. They invariably gave more significance to "freedom from symptoms with the minimum dose that will accomplish it" rather than aiming at predefined laboratory results.[33]

Preparations of thyroid extract were effective but had a disadvantage: they could not be standardized to provide uniform potency. There were major differences among the different manufacturers, even among lots from the same manufacturer. In addition, tablets containing thyroid extract were occasionally clinically inactive, most likely because of instability and reduced shelf life. Insufficient quality control in the preparation of the extracts probably explained these observations, but Hubert Richardson's book also mentions absorption issues.[34]

Thyroid extract precedes the creation of the FDA. So, its manufactures never went through a formal process of approval, and the FDA grandfathered the extract into use. Issues with inconsistent potency were the main reason physicians switched to T_4 once it was discovered that T_4 is converted to T_3 in humans; soon after, this was confirmed in many other vertebrates.

*   *   *

The first two decades after the development of thyroid extract were marked by physicians getting used to starting with small doses and slowly making adjustments based on symptoms. Once they accumulated sufficient experience, they regarded thyroid extract as an excellent treatment for hypothyroidism, only to abandon it in the 1970s and 1980s in favor of treatment with T_4.

These transitions were captured in the multiple editions of James H. Means's book *The Thyroid and Its Diseases*. In the 1937 first edition, he strongly recommends thyroid extract.[35] He carefully describes the potencies of eight different commercial brands of thyroid extract, recommending that physicians get familiar with the potency of at least two or three for their practice. His assessment did not change in the subsequent editions of his book, published in 1948 and 1963. After he died in 1967, the next edition was published in 1975. At this time, the new editors recommended treatment with either thyroid extract or T_4, saying "we prefer levothyroxine [T_4] or a mixture [of T_4 and T_3] (liotrix) as the most generally satisfactory medication, and now routinely prescribe it rather than desiccated thyroid [thyroid extract]."[36] Essentially the same recommendations were made in the 1984 edition of the book, except that the doses of both medicines were slightly reduced. Finally, the last edition of the book (1996) stated that "T_4, T_3, liotrix (combinations of T_3 and T_4), and desiccated thyroid (thyroid USP) [thyroid extract] . . . function equally well biologically, but levothyroxine [T_4] is preferred due to its long half-life [it lasts in the body for several days], its ready quantitation [measurement] in the blood, ease [of] absorption, and the availability of multiple tablet strengths."[37]

*　*　*

In the fall of 2019, I visited an industrial plant where thyroid extract is prepared. It was huge and did not smell good—as if I was locked in a butcher shop with poor ventilation. I felt transported to the set where they shot *Land of the Giants*, an old science fiction television program that aired around 1970: everything was gigantic. The equipment they used was like what I use in my laboratory, but it was made of stainless steel and it was huge, an average of fifty feet tall. The plant received daily shipments of frozen thyroid glands harvested from pigs used in the food supply, at preselected USDA-approved slaughterhouses. The manufacturers are very peculiar about their sources because the amount of T_4 and T_3 in the thyroid can change according to the weather, the soil, the season of the year, and the food given to the animals. Thus, trusting the suppliers to keep things consistent is very important.

The manufacturing of thyroid extract must comply with the Current Good Manufacturing Practice as enforced by the FDA, the failure of which may result in a product recall. In addition, companies that manufacture and commercialize thyroid extract in the United States must follow the procedures and standards described in the United States Pharmacopeia (USP).

Once the thyroids are cleaned, minced, mixed, and digested with specific enzymes and chemicals, a soup-like material is made. At each stage during the process, the soup flows through huge stainless-steel pipes, from one room to another. After the soup is centrifuged to eliminate undigested/unwanted materials, it undergoes a sterilization process, similar to pasteurization. Once the product is sterilized, it is dried and processed into a fine powder that contains T_4 and T_3. The powder is collected and shipped to another facility, where it is carefully weighed and packaged into tablets.

Thyroid extract lost its place as the leading treatment of hypothyroidism in the past mostly because of inconsistencies in the manufacturing process. Today, the USP protocol requires sophisticated measurements, and the results are then compared against their respective standards. The thyroid powder is formulated into tablets based on the amount of T_4, and the final weight is adjusted to ensure that the potency of the resulting tablet conforms with the USP recommendations, that is, a 1-grain tablet (approximately 65 milligrams) contains 38 micrograms of T_4 and 9 micrograms of T_3, with a 10% margin of error.

It is up to the manufacturers to review the data for each lot and ensure that their product meets those standards both at release and throughout its shelf life. I spoke to a representative of a large manufacturer of thyroid extract and learned that they are critically aware of the past issues with dosage and potency, which can result in voluntary drug recalls. Indeed, I keep hearing that batches of specific brands have been recalled because their content of T_4 and T_3 was outside of the expected reference range. The FDA's own website states that manufacturing and quality issues, drug recalls, and supply issues are common with medicines containing thyroid extract.[38]

*　*　*

It's amazing to me that when I was born, doctors had no way of measuring TSH levels and that patients with hypothyroidism were treated with thyroid extract. So much has changed during my lifetime in the way we treat hypothyroidism. But the changes were in the works since much earlier, when T_4 was identified as the main thyroid hormone. In the next chapter, I share the drama and excitement, plus the loneliness and the competition of this groundbreaking work in science. I also show how important collaboration and luck are to discoveries. And I demonstrate the "need" felt by doctors and scientists to know exactly what is in the thyroid extract to explain its actions. Pioneer studies in Germany and the United States gave way to no less brilliant studies done in Montreal and London until two new molecules were identified: T_4 and T_3. Doctors could now move beyond thyroid extracts and to purer, quantifiable thyroid hormones—but did they? This pressure to innovate is the context for the coming rush to a new yet not fully tested treatment.

CHAPTER 7

Pioneering a Purer Treatment

Given the success of the thyroid-extract treatments, scientists rushed to isolate the unique chemical compounds responsible for improvements seen in patients. Ultimately, they learned that two specific molecules (dubbed T_4 and T_3) are crucial to these extracts and, indeed, to those with functioning thyroids. Edward Kendall, a scientist at the Mayo Clinic in Rochester, isolated one of the molecules, T_4, and Charles Harington, at the National Institute for Medical Research (NIMR) in London, deciphered its structure. Rosalind (Ros) Pitt-Rivers and her fellow Jack Gross, also at the NIMR, isolated the other molecule.

*   *   *

Scientists purified thyroid extracts during the 1890s through different chemical techniques looking for mucin (as we saw, William Ord believed that the thyroid secretes mucin). Therefore, Charles Harington revealed in his 1933 book, *The Thyroid Gland*, that a level of surprise and disappointment came when the first purer fractions of thyroid extract did not have mucin and were not active.[1]

It was Theodor Kocher who connected the dots. He thought about the prophylactic role played by iodine in reducing goiter and in 1895 suggested that the thyroid gland might itself contain iodine. In the next year, Paul Kraske, professor of surgery at the University of Freiburg, asked Eugen Baumann, then head of the Department of Physiological Chemistry, to prepare stable preparations of the active material of the thyroid gland to treat patients. Kraske had learned of the favorable influence of thyroid substances in goiters. Baumann then processed the regular thyroid extract through a series of boiling acids and alkali, which resulted in a brownish powder that after further treatment acquired the violet color characteristic of iodine. Baumann was skeptical of Kocher's suggestion and could not believe his results. He said, "When I first made this observation, I believed in anything but that the iodine belonged to my substance."[2] He named this product thyroiodin, and later renamed it iodothyrin. The new substance was active, relieving the symptoms of thyroidectomized dogs as well as patients with hypothyroidism, and promoting considerable weight loss in obese individuals!

Baumann died prematurely, at the age of forty-nine, due to a heart problem. Others continued with the work of further characterization of iodothyrin, but it was Edward Kendall who made the most significant progress.

Kendall was destined to study the thyroid gland. After graduating from Columbia University in 1910, he worked at Parke-Davis in Detroit, where he was assigned to isolate the hormone of the thyroid gland. Unhappy with his job, he later returned to New York to work at St. Luke's Hospital, but never stopped his pursuit of the thyroid hormone.

John C. Morris, a physician-scientist at the Mayo Clinic with whom for years I had the pleasure of serving as an officer of the American Thyroid Association, is knowledgeable of Kendall's tenure at the Mayo Clinic.[3] He told me that Kendall, after learning that his request for a salary raise had been turned down in New York, applied for a position at Mayo. He was called for an interview in late 1913. With him, he brought a small vial of his most pure thyroid extract to impress his prospective employer.

It worked. William J. Mayo made him head of the Section of Biochemistry in 1914, and he was given the task of pursuing the isolation of the thyroid hormone. He was given a brand-new laboratory on the fourth floor of a recently constructed Mayo building, later known as the 1914 Building.

The Mayo Clinic had a unique interest in studies of the thyroid gland. Both Mayo brothers were surgeons and had a huge volume of patients with goiter; as we saw, surgery was needed to relieve compression symptoms in the neck. In 1908, they reported together with the endocrinologist Henry S. Plummer their experience with a thousand thyroid surgeries, and with five thousand surgeries only three years later. These are extraordinary numbers. A thyroid surgeon today is considered high-volume if they operate on more than a hundred patients a year![4]

Kendall wasted no time. On Christmas morning of the same year, he had isolated crystals of an iodine-containing substance that he named "alpha iodin." He'd been living and sleeping in the lab for days, after processing 6,500 pounds of hog thyroid. He knew he was close to isolating one of the most important components of the thyroid extract. On December 23, 1914, as the temperature outside was −6°F and snow covered the ground, Kendall had fallen asleep in the laboratory while working with thyroid extracts prepared in ethanol.

When he woke up, he saw that the ethanol had evaporated, leaving a white crusty residue surrounded by a yellow ring at the bottom of the flask. He quickly added fresh ethanol, which dissolved the yellow waxy material—but the white crust remained insoluble. He was ready to discard this crust but decided to measure its iodine content. Much to his surprise, the white crust contained about 60% iodine, which he reasoned was an indication he had isolated the main thyroid substance.

Kendall finally solubilized the white crust by using a few drops of sodium hydroxide, a common laboratory chemical. He tweaked the solution a bit more, with a strong acid this time, and crystals were formed: T_4 crystals. These were visualized through a microscope for the first time on December 25, 1914.

Following his success, Kendall immediately wanted to isolate more of the crystals. But when he tried, the result was a failure — not a partial failure, but a complete failure, he told a perplexed audience at the symposium on thyroxine to celebrate the Mayo centennial, in April 1964. A second attempt failed as well. "For a young man on his twenty-eight year, this was discouraging, frustrating, and eventually frightening," he recalled. More of the crystals were not isolated for fifteen months. He reckoned that "those in a position of authority were sympathetic and understanding."[5]

As it turns out, to scale up the isolation process, he needed sufficiently large glass flasks. He could not find them. The next best thing was a much larger tank made of galvanized iron. However, this proved to be a mistake — the galvanized iron destroyed the thyroxine molecules. He later realized that the fifteen-month hiatus was also because thyroid glands obtained during the winter contained much less thyroid hormone. When he realized his mistake and switched to large enameled kettles, he rapidly processed many hundreds of pounds of thyroids obtained from animals killed during the spring and summer, and once again obtained T_4 crystals, in August 1915.

To test if the crystals were active (if they mimic the actions of the thyroid extract), Kendall gave daily injections of 0.5 milligrams of the crystals under the skin of dogs, as well as to one child patient with cretinism and one adult with hypothyroidism. In all cases, treatment gave prompt relief of the main symptoms of overt hypothyroidism.

To figure out the chemical nature of the crystals was the next step, and probably the hardest one. Of course, Kendall did not have the formula — this was a brand-new molecule. All he knew was the work of A. Nürnberg, published a few years earlier, concluding that to make thyroid hormone iodine is combined with one of the building blocks of proteins (amino acids), either tyrosine or tryptophan. Nürnberg favored tryptophan; Kendall agreed. His analyses concluded that the newly crystalized thyroid compound was based on tryptophan combined with iodine.[6]

Tryptophan contains a structure known as an oxindole nucleus, hence, he renamed it "thyroxyindole," and then shortened it to "thyroxin." But he was wrong, and in a few years the name would have changed to *thyroxine* with an *e*. How this came about is controversial, reflecting a level of tension between Kendall and Charles Harington. Kendall realized that the building block of thyroid hormone was tyrosine and not tryptophan, which led him to rename it.[7] But his realization came through Harington's work, which started in the early 1920s. Harington's biographers indicated that renaming Kendall's crystals to *thyroxine* was Harington's suggestion.[8] Harington says in his book that "the addition ... of a terminal *e* [was] in order to conform with the British system of [chemical] nomenclature for the class of compounds to which it belongs."[9] During the 1964 Mayo Clinic Centennial Year Symposium, Pitt-Rivers had to delicately explain how Harington felt about Kendall's proposed formula to the top brass at Mayo, which also included no other than Kendall. "He concluded that there were improbabilities in Kendall's suggestion that thyroxine was an indole derivative," she explained.[10]

By 1917, Kendall had accumulated seven grams of thyroxine at $350 per gram (equivalent to $7,300 per gram today). During the next years, his work led him to propose a quasi-final chemical structure for thyroxine, but finalizing the research was delayed because of the high price of isolating its crystals. Nonetheless, he successfully patented the method to extract and crystallize thyroxine and later gave the patent as a gift to the University of Minnesota. The university negotiated a license agreement with Squibb & Sons (which eventually became the pharmaceutical Bristol Myers Squibb) and the proceeds were directed to the

Mayo Foundation for Medical Education and Research under the Kendall Thyroxin Fund. Kendall was given 10%, and his first check was cut May 16, 1929, for $252.14; his next check was for $63.28 (about $4,000 and $1,000 in today's value, respectively).

* * *

Charles Harington graduated from Cambridge University in 1919, and in 1922 earned a PhD from the University of Edinburgh. Soon after, he was appointed to the newly created post of Lecturer in Chemical Pathology at University College Hospital Medical School, London, which included the possibility of spending a year in the United States. Off he went to New York, where he worked at the Rockefeller Institute.

Perhaps due to his earlier appointment as a research assistant in the Department of Therapeutics at the Royal Infirmary, Edinburgh, where there was much interest in diseases of the thyroid gland, he became closely interested in Kendall's work. But he was increasingly dubious about the validity of Kendall's proposed structure for thyroxine (it contained only three atoms of iodine). He expressed these doubts while working with the British chemist Henry D. Dakin in New York; at Dakin's suggestion, Harington agreed, after some hesitation, to reinvestigate the structure of thyroxine when he returned to his new post in England.

Harington tried to test his ideas, but the chemical methods at that time required supplies of thyroxine in the order of ten grams. So, his first problem was to devise a more efficient method of isolation. He eventually came up with a method with a yield twenty-five times greater than that of Kendall's process. He needed cash to apply his method on a large scale. It was here that University College Hospital Medical School came to the rescue and provided him with funds to hire a commercial firm. With adequate supplies of pure thyroxine, Harington reexamined Kendall's empirical formula and, within five years, he had determined the new chemical constitution of thyroxine. He had also produced synthetic thyroxine in the laboratory from scratch.

Iodine atoms are large and heavy. For example, they weigh more than ten times what carbon atoms do, and almost 130 times what hydrogen does. That is why the four atoms of iodine play such an important role in the structure of thyroid hormone. The other atoms in the T_4 molecule are much smaller, and function as a backbone to keep the iodine atoms together, positioning them in the correct spatial architecture.

Cracking the structure of T_4 was a major achievement. Thyroxine was the first hormone to be chemically produced in a laboratory. An addendum to one of Harington's papers by his onetime Edinburgh colleague, the physician David Murray Lyon, gave the final touch to the proof that his proposed structure was right: Lyon reported that synthetic thyroxine had resolved the symptoms of two cases of overt hypothyroidism as effectively as did the crystals isolated from the hog thyroid by Kendall. It was no wonder, therefore, that when Harington communicated his results to the Biochemical Society, they were received with acclaim.

For his work on thyroid secretions, Harington was nominated for a Nobel Prize six times between 1928 and 1953, but he was overlooked each time. Kendall, on the other hand, moved on to study other molecules with hormonal activity. In 1950, Kendall received the Nobel Prize for Physiology or Medicine along with Swiss chemist Tadeusz Reichstein and Mayo Clinic physician Philip S. Hench, for their extensive work with the hormones of the adrenal gland.

*   *   *

After a long string of trials, as well as personal adventures in the lead-up to World War II, Rosalind Pitt-Rivers, with the aid of her

Canadian postdoctoral student Jack Gross, discovered in 1952 T_4's companion—originally called "unknown-1" by Gross and Charles Leblond, but later recognized as T_3.

Pitt-Rivers belonged to an aristocratic family. Her interest in chemistry began at the age of twelve, when her uncle gave her a chemistry set.[11] She married her cousin, Captain George Henry Lane Fox Pitt-Rivers, the grandson of the archaeologist who founded the Pitt Rivers Museum at Oxford. He was an anthropologist and eugenicist who was one of the wealthiest men in England in the interwar period. One year later they had a son, but their marriage rapidly deteriorated as her husband had become increasingly pro-eugenics and antisemitic, drawing closer to German eugenicists and praising Mussolini and Hitler. She left the Pitt-Rivers estate in 1937, her departure soon to be followed by acrimonious divorce; by 1940, George Pitt-Rivers was interned in the Tower of London.[12]

The divorce brought her back to science, and in the autumn of 1937, she joined Harington at University College Hospital Medical School in London. One of her son's earliest memories is of his mother simultaneously reading to him, knitting, and smoking.[13] She worked for her doctoral degree under Albert Nurnberger in Harington's Department of Biochemistry and obtained a PhD in biochemistry in 1939.

Pitt-Rivers joined Harington's group and moved with him in 1941 to the NIMR as a member of the Medical Research Council's scientific staff. But World War II disrupted her career progression. She played significant roles in the war effort; toward the end of the war, she was deployed with the army to Belgium, where she assisted the nutrition (reintroduction of food for malnourished or starving individuals needs to be done thoughtfully) in prisoners of concentration camps. With the end of the war, she returned to NIMR and vigorously resumed her studies.

Pitt-Rivers was curious about the potency of the thyroid secretion and the fact that there was a delay of several hours after

T_4 administration before effects could be detected. She considered that T_4 was metabolized before it could trigger effects in the body. Indeed, her career was permeated by the search and characterization of thyroid-hormone metabolites. In this regard, she followed with interest the work being done at McGill University in Montreal by Jack Gross, a young physician working toward his PhD under the mentorship of Charles Leblond, an imaging expert at McGill who invented autoradiography (a method to visualize radioactive molecules by exposure to photographic emulsions).

For his thesis, Gross injected rats with radioactive iodine. As we saw, iodine is normally trapped in the thyroid and used to make thyroid hormones. And so is radioactive iodine. After a few hours, Gross killed the rats and analyzed their thyroids for the presence of radioactive molecules. He knew the thyroid gland of the rat would take up radioactive iodine to make T_4, so he was not surprised when he saw that the majority of the radioactive molecules was simply T_4. However, he also observed the presence of an unknown radioactive molecule, which he named unknown-1.

In the autumn of 1950, Gross then moved to the NIMR as a postdoctoral fellow at the Pitt-Rivers laboratory (now relocated to Mill Hill, a suburb in the London borough of Barnet). His most pressing priority was to identify unknown-1. Pitt-Rivers's expertise in organic chemistry proved invaluable in this task. Having a hunch that unknown-1 could be T_3, she immediately set to work to produce T_3 in the laboratory. Then Pitt-Rivers and Gross studied both molecules side by side, and soon proved that the synthetic, crystalline T_3 was identical to unknown-1. Their findings were published in the prestigious journal *Lancet* and were followed by two more publications in that same journal (one showing in rats that T_3 was more potent than synthetic T_4, and the other that T_3 could reverse the effects of hypothyroidism in humans, the latter with the help of Wilfred R. Trotter, a consultant physician at the University College Hospital in London).[14]

It is interesting that in a series of correspondences with Clark Sawin, the clinician-scientist at the Boston VA hospital, Pitt-Rivers describes Harington's lukewarm reaction upon learning about T_3 being unknown-1: "Oh, how disappointing"—perhaps thinking that T_3 was a weaker breakdown product of T_4. Later, after learning that T_3 was three to four times more potent than T_4, he was overcome with surprise. The news contradicted his long-held belief that T_4 was the legitimate thyroid hormone.[15]

Like Kendall, Pitt-Rivers also faced stiff competition, which made those days in late 1951 and early 1952 very exciting for them. They worked long into the night, seven days a week. They knew that the team at the Collège de France in Paris, including Serge Lissitzky, Raymond Michel, and Jean Roche, was hot on the same trail. Indeed, that team independently identified T_3 in the thyroid gland at about the same time. It is revealing of Pitt-Rivers's character that, despite their sharp scientific rivalry, she and Michel remained lifelong friends and later collaborated.

*　*　*

Once the structures for T_4 and T_3 were resolved and both molecules could be made in the laboratory, pharmaceutical companies jumped in. They rushed to prepare medicinal grades of both molecules, making them available to treat patients with hypothyroidism. However, thyroid extracts were so effective that physicians used T_4 and T_3 only sparsely, not understanding them very well. Each molecule was seen as an independent hormone produced by the thyroid gland. Whereas both hormones reproduced the metabolic actions of thyroid secretion, there were noticeable differences when either was used individually to treat patients with hypothyroidism.

Thus, during the next twenty years, neither T_4 nor T_3 achieved a dominant position as the treatment of choice for hypothyroidism; thyroid extract remained the standard of care. T_4 was seen as a slow-acting molecule with more prolonged effects than natural thyroid secretions or thyroid extract. Conversely, the actions of T_3 exhibited rapid onset but brief duration, producing brisk but short-lived clinical changes.

Only after scientists in Boston and New York unequivocally demonstrated that T_4 is converted to T_3 in patients with hypothyroidism, did treatment with T_4 gain momentum.

* * *

It is fascinating to see how the quest to identify the hormones in thyroid extract ping-ponged between Freiburg, Rochester, and London, whereas that of T_3 started in Montreal and ended almost at the same time in London and in Paris. The next chapter closes the history section of the book, by bringing you up to the present day. In it, I detail the story of the discovery that T_4 is converted to T_3 and how this finding was subsequently retracted, only to be rediscovered some fifteen years later.

The next chapter also contains one of the major revelations, and arguments, of the book: that in rushing forward, the medical establishment and the pharmaceutical industry never reckoned with the consequences of their change of view. The new treatments were—and are—effective. But they had substantial percentages of failures, which left some patients worse off than when they were on their treatments with thyroid extract. Here is the moment when doctors not only promoted a new, perhaps a less effective treatment, but it is the moment they began ignoring data, and brushing off those patients who voiced concerns.

CHAPTER 8

Dangers of Untested Treatments

Despite tremendous scientific progress toward understanding the thyroid gland and its hormones, up until the 1960s and 1970s there were no objective methods with sufficient specificity to diagnose hypothyroidism and to adjust the dose of thyroid extract. The disease continued to be diagnosed and managed clinically, based on signs and symptoms, as it was done almost a century earlier. Treatment was still based on daily tablets containing an extract of pig thyroid. This was good but not perfect, and issues such as variable shelf life and unreliable potency remained in the minds of the physicians.

Physicians started treatment with a small dose, adjusting it very slowly, according to how the patient was feeling. However, the line that separated "feeling well" from "feeling jittery" was a thin one. Patients could easily be given too much thyroid extract, which causes palpitations—a sensation of a fast heartbeat—as well as chest pain, headaches, and tremor. Speaking with my colleagues who practiced at that time, signs of excessive treatment were not easy to determine, particularly in older adults. One of the first signs was a fine tremor in the hands, which was not uncommon and indicated the dose of extract had to be lowered or stopped until symptoms were eliminated.

The development of TSH testing occurred in the mid- to late

1960s, and its clinical availability in the early 1970s constituted the most accurate way of assessing the functioning of the thyroid gland. The discovery that T_4 is converted to T_3 in human tissues outside the thyroid gland occurred in 1970.[1] The interpretation at the time was that this discovery obviated the need of treating patients with thyroid extract, which contains both T_4 and T_3.

As a result, treatment switched, but with unforeseen consequences. Carefully adjusted doses of T_4 replaced thyroid extract, at doses calibrated to normalize circulating levels of TSH, not to alleviate symptoms. While most patients felt fine, some rejected the new treatment right away. According to my colleagues who were practicing at that time, many patients refused the new treatment and asked to be placed back on thyroid extract.[2]

Despite some resistance, this change in the way patients were treated was so well introduced and accepted by physicians that within the next ten years, by 1980, they all but abandoned the use of thyroid extract. The pharmaceutical grade of T_4 took its place, identical to the one isolated from hog's thyroid so many years ago by Edward Kendall on a Christmas morning. Sold under the brand name Synthroid (as well as others), synthetic T_4 became the standard of care for hypothyroidism.

*   *   *

For several years, scientists knew that TSH is a hormone that controls the thyroid gland and that TSH levels fluctuate inversely with the activity of the gland. However, a robust method for measuring TSH levels in the blood that could be used clinically was not available. I had the privilege of working for almost ten years in the office next door to the man who developed such a method. During those years, Robert (Bob) D. Utiger served in the editorial office of the *New England Journal of Medicine* and other medical journals, where he used his red pen to provide prospective authors with extensive feedback after they thought they had the "final" version of the manuscript.

In the early 1960s, Utiger worked at the Endocrinology Branch of the NIH as a physician-scientist, where he studied antibodies against TSH. This work served as the basis for his landmark publication in 1965 on a novel method to measure TSH levels in the blood. A few years earlier, Rosalyn Yalow, a scientist at the VA hospital in the Bronx, had developed a method known as radioimmunoassay to measure hormones in the blood, for which she won the Nobel Prize in Physiology or Medicine in 1977. The method required good antibodies directed against the hormone being measured. Given its success, such methods were pouring forth throughout the field, so Utiger wasted no time using his antibodies against TSH to set up a test for TSH that could be used clinically.

In subsequent years, Utiger's original method was improved to allow the measurement of progressively smaller amounts of TSH in the blood, and today we have what is called an ultrasensitive assay. The test to measure TSH levels is still one of the most frequently used in medicine because of its utility in the diagnosis of thyroid diseases. Its normal reference range in the blood is between 0.45 and 4.5 µU/ml, but in hypothyroid patients, it can frequently reach values between 10 and 100 µU/ml. (See chapter 1.)

Measuring circulating-TSH levels turned out to be the most sensitive and specific method to diagnose hypothyroidism, rising rapidly to become the standard of care a few years after its inception. The importance of measuring TSH to diagnose hypothyroidism cannot be overstated. This method changed what had been practiced for ninety years—no longer were physicians diagnosing hypothyroidism based on symptoms, signs, and laboratory parameters that lacked sensitivity and specificity.

The clinical utilization of TSH to diagnose hypothyroidism was so obvious that almost immediately, physicians also started using TSH levels in the circulation to evaluate patients with hypothyroidism kept on thyroid extract. They expected that those patients feeling good on thyroid extract would also exhibit normal TSH levels. In other words, a TSH within normal range would indicate that the amount of thyroid hormones provided by the daily tablets of thyroid extract was sufficient, equivalent to what a normal thyroid gland produced daily.

However, the results surprised physicians. They saw that patients doing well on thyroid extract had TSH levels well below normal range, sometimes undetectable. They were being given much more thyroid extract than necessary to normalize TSH levels. That meant that the dose of thyroid extract that resolved the symptoms of hypothyroidism and made patients feel well was way above the dose needed to normalize circulating levels of TSH. This led physicians to progressively reduce the dose of thyroid extract based on TSH levels, independently of how a patient was feeling.

Unfortunately, as physicians were also abandoning thyroid extract in favor of synthetic thyroid hormones, there was no opportunity or interest in accumulating experience with the use of thyroid extract monitored with TSH levels. In retrospect, it is hard to say exactly why this happened, but it was likely due to a combination of a bad reputation for thyroid extract (being inconsistent) and excitement with the new approach involving T_4.

In our minds, a patient should feel well once the TSH level returns to normal. In addition, physicians are well aware that too much thyroid extract could cause adverse reactions. Thus, normalizing TSH levels while avoiding these symptoms was considered a plus and became the standard of care.

* * *

With the discovery and knowledge of the molecular structures of T_4 and T_3, physicians were taking steps toward clarifying their role in the treatment of hypothyroidism. T_4 and T_3 became commercially available in the 1950s, and each exhibited metabolic actions similar to the body's thyroid hormones. At Johns Hopkins University in Baltimore, Samuel P. Asper was a superb clinical investigator focused on thyroid diseases. Around 1954, he and his fellow Herbert Selenkow treated six hypothyroid patients with T_3 for several weeks and then switched them to T_4. They studied the patients on either treatment and made two important observations.[3]

First, either T_4 alone or T_3 alone eliminated symptoms of hypothyroidism. However, both treatments failed to restore the blood levels of PBI, an index of the amount of iodine bound to proteins in the blood, commonly used by physicians at the time to estimate the amounts of thyroid hormones in the blood. Treatment with T_4 made PBI levels too high, and treatment with T_3 made them too low. Physicians were confused by this because a high PBI traditionally meant hyperthyroidism and a low PBI meant hypothyroidism. How could the patients have such disparate PBI levels and feel fine?

Second, the clinical and metabolic properties of T_3 are qualitatively identical to those of T_4 and thyroid extract. Therefore, they reasoned that the synthetic compounds were advantageous, mainly because they avoided fluctuations in hormonal potency (as observed with thyroid extract).

Despite these encouraging results, the apparent disconnect between the resolution of symptoms and PBI levels confused physicians. Thus, even with the commercial availability of T_4 and T_3, thyroid extract remained the standard of care to treat hypothyroidism, as it contained a mixture of T_4 and T_3.

Following his fellowship, Selenkow was recruited by the Peter Bent Brigham Hospital, where he remained for the next four decades. He was brought to Boston initially to begin the Thyroid Laboratory, where he served as director from 1956 to 1975 (succeeded by Reed Larsen). Selenkow was a great mentor to his fellows, and together they conducted several studies, mostly on hyperthyroidism (Graves' disease). But he kept in the back of his mind the studies he had initiated with Asper at Hopkins, comparing T_4 and T_3. Then, in 1964, he decided to resume those studies. He had a young fellow working with him, Marvin S. Wool.

Wool considered Selenkow a brilliant scientist and followed his lead. Selenkow's motivation to do the studies was to define how best to achieve physiological supplementation of thyroid hormones. They asked their lab assistant, Victor Fang, to carefully grind up tablets of T_4 and T_3 to a fine powder, mix them at different ratios, and repackage the mixture in capsules. They recruited twenty-one patients with hypothyroidism, who were treated with either T_4 or T_3, but also with the capsules containing different ratios of $T_4 + T_3$. (Preparing the capsules was labor intensive—Wool remembers Fang spending much of his day grinding those tablets. By the time the study was ongoing and they obtained preliminary results, they were able to convince a pharmaceutical company to assist with the preparation of the rest of the capsules.)

After studying several metabolic parameters, Selenkow and Wool concluded that the optimal treatment was a combination of approximately 175 micrograms of T_4 and 50 micrograms of T_3 (a 3.5:1 ratio). The mixture had the clinical advantage of mimicking all the metabolic effects of normal thyroid-hormone secretions while producing normal PBI levels in the circulation.

These findings led to the idea that T_4 and T_3 complement each other in the treatment of hypothyroidism, and only their combination could eliminate symptoms and restore PBI *at the same time*. Hence was born the idea that thyroid-hormone supplementation had to be made with combinations of T_4 and T_3 to treat patients with hypothyroidism.

The results were so powerful and so convincing that Forest Laboratories decided to market liotrix, a mixture of synthetic

$T_4 + T_3$ (4:1), that was formulated to treat hypothyroidism. The FDA approved liotrix for the treatment of hypothyroidism (Thyrolar) in December 1969.

However, just six months later, in May 1970, physician-scientists in Boston and New York forever changed the thyroid world, showing T_4-to-T_3 conversion in humans.[4] As we have seen, physicians interpreted this to mean there was no need to treat patients with T_3, just T_4. As a result, liotrix, created to eliminate the inconsistency issues with thyroid extract, never took off. There were a couple of studies published in France, but never a clinical trial comparing liotrix with T_4.

This was a major missed opportunity, a turning point in the story of combination therapy. Had the gap between the FDA approval of liotrix and the discovery of T_4-to-T_3 conversion been wider, physicians would have acquired experience monitoring its use with TSH testing, and things could have been much different. During the subsequent years, the commercial availability of liotrix was spotty, until finally, its maker, Allergan, pulled it off the market.

Marvin Wool went on to private practice, where until a few years ago he saw thousands of patients with hypothyroidism. He never prescribed combination therapy. Despite his pivotal work with Selenkow, he remained fully convinced that T_4 at doses that normalize TSH levels resolves all symptoms. "It was very convenient to have all those tablets with multiple doses of T_4 to adjust TSH levels," he said when I spoke to him in the summer of 2021.

*　　*　　*

With T_3's identification in the early 1950s, the relationship between T_4 and T_3 took multiple turns. Jack Gross and Ros Pitt-Rivers remained curious about the fact that T_4 had a delay of several hours or even days to function, and kept thinking that the time was needed for the body to modify the T_4 molecule in a way that triggered its effects. Given that the difference between T_4 and T_3 is one iodine atom only, right from the start they wondered whether the thyroid or other organs could activate T_4 simply by removing this iodine atom and whether this would reflect a natural process. Gross and Leblond had obtained early evidence that this is indeed the case.[5] And so did Edwin Albright, a physician at the University of Wisconsin in 1954, and his colleagues.[6] So, it seems that around that time, momentum was building to recognize that T_4-to-T_3 conversion was part of the normal functioning of the thyroid system.

*　　*　　*

Jack Gross left Mill Hill to become a professor of histology at SUNY Downstate College of Medicine, and Pitt-Rivers embarked on a search for T_3 analogs (T_3-like molecules) that were even more potent or more rapid. This coincided with her decision to spend a sabbatical year abroad, between 1953 and 1954. She came to Boston and worked with John Stanbury, a clinician-scientist head of the Thyroid Unit at Mass General Hospital at the time. Stanbury started his career in medical practice and endocrine research in the thyroid lab at Mass General. His passion was the thyroid and how iodine deficiency leads to goiter, at the time still a widespread condition around the world. He ultimately demonstrated the link between reduced dietary iodine and intellectual disability and neurological deficits and went on to become a world advocate for the addition of iodine to salt in countries with inadequate dietary iodine, as told in his 2008 book, *The Iodine Trail*.[7]

I met Stanbury a few times and spoke with him at length at a gathering at Reed Larsen's house. He was a tall, heavily built man, who had served in the navy for four years during World War II. He told me that in the 1950s, he flew to Argentina and explored the cities near the Andes looking for individuals with goiter. His heavy equipment, such as Geiger counters and scanners, were transported by ship from Boston and then flown to the Andes. They flew the radioactive iodine directly from the United States to be used for the first time in the country.

It was during that sabbatical year in Boston that Pitt-Rivers obtained solid evidence of T_4-to-T_3 conversion in humans. She and Stanbury treated six hypothyroid patients with radioactive T_4 (similar to what Gross and Leblond had done with rodents) and, remarkably, identified small amounts of radioactive T_3 in the blood of these patients. After T_4 administration, the T_3 levels in the blood increased rapidly and peaked about twenty hours later. The data presented in their publication is very convincing.[8]

However, like Charles Harington, Stanbury believed firmly that T_4 was the key hormone produced by the thyroid and wasn't sure the conversion to T_3 reflected a necessary pathway involved in the actions of thyroid hormones. It could be, for example, that T_4 was transformed to T_3 as the first step of its elimination from the body. In addition, he wondered if the technique used to identify T_3 was sensitive enough.

Stanbury's biggest concern was the spontaneous conversion of T_4 to T_3 that could occur during the time needed to separate and identify T_3. Adding to these technical concerns, Pitt-Rivers was unimpressed with T_3 as a key physiological molecule because its effects were so short lived; she thought that perhaps other modifications in either the T_4 or the T_3 molecule could be more physiologically relevant.

As both Stanbury and Pitt-Rivers remained skeptical about the physiological role of deiodination (the conversion of T_4 to T_3), in 1958, Stanbury retracted their paper! He repeated the experiments using an alternative method, descending paper chromatography, which provided better separation of T_4 and T_3 and was unable to confirm their previous work.[9]

Years later, in a 1962 interview, Pitt-Rivers said that the idea that T_4 was not active until it had been converted to T_3, was just a hypothesis that had been floated by Jack Gross and her when they discovered T_3. She recalled when in 1959 she was visiting the NIH and picked up a physiology book from a library table, and in that book, she read "the astonishing statement that thyroxine is no longer believed to be the thyroid hormone." She shivered at the idea that their past remark, meant to be a challenge to the field, had been jumped upon and converted to a fact in a textbook. "One wonders how long will it take to remove this out of the textbooks," she said, and the audience laughed. She gave a few reasons for why it would not make sense for T_4 to be activated to T_3. But she never mentioned her 1955 work with Stanbury showing T_4-to-T_3 conversion in humans. It seems that in her mind, she wrote that off after the retraction.[10]

* * *

Sidney (Sid) Ingbar was a physician-scientist at the Beth Israel Hospital in Boston. He was a world-class authority on the thyroid gland and its diseases, well known for his work on how proteins in the blood are attached to thyroid hormones. I interacted very little with Ingbar during my time in Boston, but distinctly remember him standing by the door talking to his fellows, as he could not step into the laboratory while smoking. He was charismatic and attracted scientists from all over the world—more than a hundred younger associates in all, many of whom have become academic leaders in the United States, Europe, South America, North Africa, and Asia.

Ingbar recognized the Beth Israel intern Lew Braverman's value and immediately engaged him in his studies. Indeed, Braverman became a physician-scientist, a giant in endocrinology, and a renowned leader in the thyroid field. Braverman and Ingbar worked together for several years, and they were friends.

David, Ingbar's eldest son, has fresh memories of those days. On weekends the house always had either fellows, trainees, or Braverman coming over. And they wrote manuscripts on yellow legal pads, cutting and pasting and scratching, while there was some sort of sports game on half the time. As a teenager, David remembers a glowing, positive atmosphere of constant excitement about science.

Ingbar was known for thinking outside the box. He enjoyed pursuing unconventional ideas; in the late 1960s, they decided to revisit the physiological relevance of T_4 activation to T_3 in humans. His interest in the subject may have been sparked earlier. In 1956 he spent a sabbatical year in London working in Pitt-Rivers's laboratory, where Val Galton was a doctoral student. Surely they talked about deiodination, eventually formulating the hypothesis that the actions of T_4 were linked to how it is metabolized—in particular, deiodination. A few years later, Galton came to Boston as the Milton research fellow in Ingbar's laboratory and further explored these concepts. They studied T_4 metabolism and action in bullfrogs, but could not get a pulse on the physiological phenomenon they were chasing.[11]

Only later did Ingbar approach the issue again, this time in humans, with Lew Braverman. They studied thirteen patients with hypothyroidism being treated with Synthroid (T_4). To their surprise, they found substantial amounts of T_3 in the circulation of all thirteen patients. They also collaborated with Kenneth Sterling, a nuclear medicine physician at Columbia-Presbyterian Medical Center in New York, and performed similar studies as done by Gross, Leblond, and Pitt-Rivers. They administered radioactive T_4 to these patients and successfully detected radioactive T_3 in their system.[12]

David went off to college in 1970, but he remembers (those last couple of years that led to their pivotal discovery) his dad and Braverman talking about the study and following those patients, and seeing what was happening, with an aura of great excitement—they knew they had found something really special. They took these findings as conclusive evidence that T_4 could be converted to T_3 in humans. These results were published in May 1970 and once again renewed the prospect that T_4 could be used in the treatment of hypothyroidism.

*   *   *

Lew Braverman had a big heart and loved children. Around 2003, I was in an airplane going to a thyroid conference in Florida with my triplets, who were two years old at the time. I was in the back of the plane, having a hard time with my daughter. She would not stop crying. He heard the commotion, came from the front cabin, and picked up Laura; within a minute, she was silent, sleeping.

In 2012, while I was chief of endocrinology at the University of Miami, Braverman visited with us. He gave a superb lecture on the effects of iodine on the thyroid, and later we had dinner with the fellows. They were fascinated by him. Later he surprised me with a thank-you card that he mailed instead of e-mailing. I keep it inside one of his books.

*   *   *

In September 1970, the same year Sterling published with Braverman and Ingbar, he also published another study showing T_4-to-T_3 conversion in healthy individuals with a normal thyroid gland. This time the volunteers received intravenous injections of radioactive T_4 daily for ten consecutive days before the levels of radioactive T_3 were measured. All these studies put to rest any doubt that the conversion of T_4 to T_3 is part of normal human physiology.[13]

A few years later, Jack Oppenheimer and his colleagues at

Montefiore Medical Center discovered that for thyroid hormone to act in the body, it exits the bloodstream and enters different organs where it binds to a receptor.[14] They also discovered that the molecule of thyroid hormone that is mostly attracted by the receptor is T_3 and not T_4! This finding, combined with the knowledge that T_4 is transformed to T_3, confirmed the idea that T_4 is a prohormone (with little activity) and T_3 is the main thyroid hormone responsible for the activity of thyroid secretion. Only after T_4 is converted to T_3 is the full effect of thyroid secretion released through the body.

These were indeed very important discoveries, as they carried significant clinical implications. The immediate consequence of these findings was that synthetic T_4 could be used to treat hypothyroid patients if given at the right dose. T_4 would be absorbed into the circulation and attracted to organs where the powerful T_3 molecule would be produced. (Again, this process is known as deiodination, or, simply, removal of an atom of iodine.) Physicians and scientists assumed at the time that normal amounts of T_3 would be produced. The fact that T_4 is a weaker molecule and is only slowly transformed to the active T_3, minimized the chances of overtreatment and undesirable symptoms.

* * *

From a medical perspective, the new approach to treat hypothyroidism with T_4 made perfect sense. It reflected the successful progress toward understanding the mechanisms regulating the thyroid gland. It also allowed physicians to replace the less reliable thyroid extract with T_4, a molecule that could be administered with a much higher level of accuracy, precision, and reliability. Lastly, treating hypothyroid patients with T_4 had the advantage of not causing side effects (such as palpitations, sweating, and tremor commonly observed when treatment included the powerful molecule T_3 or thyroid extract). This is because T_4 is a weaker molecule and is only slowly transformed to the active T_3.

But the assumption that T_4 was superior was never formally tested in a clinical trial that compared T_4 with thyroid extract. The switch was based both on common sense and on reports that treatment with T_4 normalizes TSH levels and resolves symptoms of overt hypothyroidism, such as cold intolerance, constipation, puffiness under the eyes, and weight gain. These studies included a very small number of patients and did not investigate quality of life, mood, or cognitive function. As I mentioned, almost immediately after the switch, it became clear that the new treatment was not as effective to resolve all symptoms of hypothyroidism. Some patients on T_4 controlled with TSH complained of residual symptoms including "foggy brain," memory impairment, poor motivation, and low energy. These were the exact symptoms described by my two patients in Miami (see chapter 1).

Selwyn Taylor, the surgeon-scientist at Hammersmith Hospital in London, provided scientific documentation of this effect in 1970. In the United States, supporting evidence was published in the early 1980s by Clark Sawin, the clinician-scientist at the Boston VA hospital. He and his colleagues identified about 120 older adults that were part of the Framingham Heart Study and were found to be on thyroid extract. In subsequent years, these patients had the opportunity to switch to T_4 but, by the time they were reanalyzed seven years later, ninety patients remained on thyroid extract.[15]

I saw this firsthand for many years. Now and then I would invariably be asked to see a patient on thyroid extract or combination therapy. My immediate reaction was to take these patients off these medications and place them on T_4. It would take a long time and some effort to explain that the body converts T_4 to T_3, which obviated the use of thyroid extract or T_3. Their response was almost always the same: thank you, but no thank you.

From a retired state senator who flew to Chicago to see me to a woman inmate in Dade County Jail, the answer was always a categorical no. Both were on astronomical doses of T_3 when I first saw them, despite their marked differences in socioeconomic status and lifestyle. As with any other such patients, they said that many doctors before me had tried the same thing. In general, these patients stress that they cannot bear to live on T_4 alone, mainly because of fatigue and difficulty focusing. Some tried for a few weeks or even months after my insistence, but invariably demanded the old therapy. As my understanding of the disease evolved, I gave up trying to have them switch. For all patients younger than sixty-five, I would just make sure the TSH levels were within normal range and refill their prescriptions.

* * *

We've covered the most important aspects of the history of hypothyroidism and thyroid hormones. The next part of the book is eye-opening—it is the core of the book. I admit that up until about ten years ago I wasn't aware of the evidence you are about to see. With a sense of awe, I learned what my colleagues had already discovered years earlier about patients with residual symptoms of hypothyroidism. It is remarkable the many ways these symptoms have been documented in the 10–20% minority that suffer.

In the next part, I also discuss how work done in my laboratory shines a spotlight on "TSH dogma," which ignores the fact that T_4-treated patients with hypothyroidism maintain relatively lower blood levels of T_3. While this could explain some of their residual symptoms, there is more to it—much more.

PART FOUR

The Patients

CHAPTER 9

Those Left Behind

In the late 1980s, Colin Dayan, a clinician-scientist at Cardiff University School of Medicine in Wales faced increasingly unhappy patients. He had recently started "fine-tuning" their T_4 doses, using TSH levels rather than symptoms in the adjustment.

Dayan was puzzled by his patients' reactions, but he was not alone. David Carr, a physician in North Tees General Hospital, Cleveland, in England had to increase the doses of T_4 to above what was required to normalize TSH levels, in order to see the patients' self-assessment scores improve. This suggested that the optimal dose of T_4—as defined by TSH levels—was insufficient to eliminate all symptoms.[1]

These observations occurred at the end of a transition period during which T_4 replaced thyroid extract as a treatment for hypothyroidism, and when the use of TSH monitoring became established practice to adjust the dose of T_4. Dayan worried because the number of unhappy patients kept increasing.

*　*　*

Years later, in the spring of 1996, Naomi Roberts at Barrow Hospital, also in England, was seeing that a surprising number of her patients had thyroid diseases. She wrote an open letter explaining what she was seeing and asking readers about psychological problems they had experienced while suffering from thyroid diseases. By the end of that summer, Roberts had received 118 letters.[2]

Several people wrote about their relief to discover that other people had felt as strange as they did. Roberts summarized her findings: many people found their doctors "unsympathetic," and these doctors were often referring patients to psychiatrists. Thirty-four people mentioned that they had not felt "normal" despite their thyroid function being in the typical range. Many were depressed and worried about how their illness affected other members of the family.

Out of seventy-four letters from patients with hypothyroidism, fifty-six mentioned memory difficulties. Letters also described difficulties concentrating, making decisions, and thinking clearly. Several people had noticed that they had trouble finding the right word to use just when they needed it. This was a particularly difficult problem for several teachers who wrote letters—standing up in front of a class of students, they were left baffled and confused. Reading about these teachers makes me think of my two patients in Miami who could no longer continue with their jobs. Thyroid problems affected a wide variety of everyday activities: driving, counting out money, spelling, cooking, sewing, completing crosswords, and writing (letters, essays, and in one case poetry).

Around the same time, John Lazarus, a clinician-scientist also in Wales, published an opinion piece saying that, in his experience, normalization of the T_3 levels in the circulation and recovery of all symptoms of hypothyroidism were achieved only with complete suppression of TSH levels, which of course required slightly higher doses of T_4.[3] But Lazarus noted that in some patients this was the only way to eliminate all symptoms.

* * *

In 1997, Jean-Jacques Staub, a clinician-scientist in Basel, Switzerland, examined and interviewed about seventy T_4-treated patients with normal TSH levels along with about one hundred "controls," patients with no thyroid disease.[4] He did not observe any differences between both groups. This was in sharp contrast to the experiences in Wales, but his tests and interviews addressed only classic signs and symptoms of overt hypothyroidism, such as dry skin, constipation, cold intolerance, hoarseness, face puffiness. His studies did not address aspects of cognition, mood, or behavior.

Dayan, back in Cardiff, saw an opportunity. He assembled a team and designed a study to address this critical void. They knew this was a difficult area to research: many of the symptoms of hypothyroidism are nonspecific and can be confused with low mood, stress-related illness, or depression due to other causes. Both depressed mood and T_4 supplementation are common conditions in the general population. Thus, a causal relationship between them could easily be wrongly inferred.

Nonetheless, the team felt that the rising concern over the issue of T_4 supplementation among patient support groups was pressing. There was a critical need to investigate the possibility that some patients were receiving inadequate thyroid hormones despite circulating-TSH levels in normal range.

Dayan and his team combed through the records of five general practices in an area of southwest England covering a population of sixty-three thousand. They identified almost a thousand adult patients who had been taking T_4 for at least four months. They also identified control subjects from the same practices with the same age and sex as each of the patients.

All these individuals were sent two questionnaires by mail. The first was a general health questionnaire asking patients to describe how they currently felt compared with their normal expectations. The second was a thyroid symptom questionnaire, derived from the symptoms reported by Naomi Roberts's patients.

The results of their study were published in October 2002.[5] They received the responses of about four hundred patients who had normal TSH levels. In these questionnaires, high scores on a scale of 1 through 4 indicate more symptoms. The number of individuals scoring 3 or more on general health was 49% in the T_4-treated patients, as opposed to 26% in the control individuals. These differences in scores remained even after matching for age, sex, and the presence of other chronic diseases.

The importance of this study cannot be overstated. For the first time and based on a scientific approach, it became clear that a substantial number of patients with hypothyroidism appropriately treated with T_4 remained symptomatic—and had lower scores on quality-of-life questionnaires when compared to a general population.

* * *

Soon doctors were sounding the alarms on the Continent as well—this time in the Netherlands. At the University of Amsterdam, Wilmar Wiersinga, a well-rounded clinician-scientist with extensive experience in thyroid diseases, decided to take on this problem. I frequently see Wiersinga at conferences, but several years ago I had a chance to chat with him at length and learn more about his work while both of us were in Paris for a few days. We were representing our thyroid societies, European and American, in the committee that prepared the program for the International Thyroid Congress in Paris in 2010.

Alerted by Roberts's and Dayan's work in the United Kingdom and by what his patients were telling him, Wiersinga wasted no time. He obtained research funds and initiated studies around the year 2000 to explore improvements in the treatment of hypothyroidism, focusing on cognitive function in these patients.[6]

Wiersinga and his colleagues acknowledged that although hormonal supplementation therapy had been successful in reducing symptoms of overt hypothyroidism, their clinical practice experience indicated that some patients had persistent symptoms, despite adequate treatment with T_4. These symptoms were vague and nonspecific, about fatigue, muscle aches, depressed mood, or decreased memory function. The doctors were aware of scattered reports based on a few patients, indicating that treatment of hypothyroidism with T_4 could be associated with only partial recovery of overall neurocognitive functioning. Hence, they wondered whether this was what they were seeing in their offices.

To tackle that problem, Wiersinga cooperated with psychiatrists at his institution. This is how he encountered Ellie Wekking, at that time a registered neuropsychologist. She oversaw the cognitive tests. These are not only quite time-consuming but also require a great deal of skill and understanding to be applied properly. She also supervised a couple of junior doctors and psychologists on how to perform these tests and apply the well-being questionnaires.

Wilmar and his colleagues recruited about 140 adult T_4-treated patients from thirteen general practices in the cities of Amsterdam and Almere. At these practices, prescribing records were checked to identify all patients receiving T_4 treatment. They all had Hashimoto's disease (the autoimmune disease that destroys the thyroid gland), had been treated for at least six months, and had a normal TSH level.

For the study, patients arrived in the morning while fasting, and after blood sampling, they took their usual dose of T_4 and had breakfast. About one hour later they proceeded with the cognitive testing session that lasted about an hour and a half and handed over the baseline set of questionnaires they had filled out on the day before the visit. These were used to assess well-being—mental health and vitality. Overall, patients went through a series of complex memory and attention tests.

The study revealed that patients with hypothyroidism appropriately maintained on T_4 performed worse when compared with the reference population. They also exhibited a lower mean level of general well-being, as well as a lower level of health-related quality of life. These findings were published in December 2005. They confirmed and expanded the findings obtained in the United Kingdom a few years earlier.

* * *

In the early 1990s, Oregon Health & Science University in Portland recruited Mary Samuels as a clinician-scientist. She had trained with E. Chester (Chip) Ridgway, a physician-scientist at the University of Colorado, and wanted to develop a clinical thyroid group to study hypothyroidism. During her training, she became aware that some patients with hypothyroidism remained symptomatic despite being appropriately treated with T_4; her mentor Ridgway was fully aware as well (and so were most endocrinologists at the time). But neither considered these symptoms as a treatment failure. Very few people did at the time. They thought that many other reasons could explain the symptoms. Just like most of us did, Samuels would just assure such patients that the symptoms were unrelated to hypothyroidism.

While she was setting up shop at the new place, she collaborated with two established local investigators, Jeri Janowsky, an expert in cognition, aging, and brain development, and Jonathan Purnell, an endocrinologist with experience in metabolism. Through these collaborations, Samuels learned a lot about the approaches and tools used by these investigators. Soon, she realized that she could use her acquired knowledge and the new tools to study patients with subclinical hypothyroidism—patients with no symptoms who have mildly elevated TSH but normal T_4 and T_3 levels.

Samuels was aware that bias is a powerful interference in studies of mood, cognition, and quality of life. For example, being diagnosed (labeled) and treated for hypothyroidism—a chronic disease—is sufficient to negatively impact the responses in those questionnaires. Thus, she wanted to develop a model to avoid this interference, which eventually she did, but the study she designed involved many patients and was expensive.

To obtain funding, she used a two-step approach. First, she obtained seed money from a foundation and performed a much smaller pilot study. Once she did this, she then used the results from the pilot study to apply for a full grant from the NIH, which would fund the expensive study. The strategy paid off.

With the seed money, she studied twenty healthy individuals and thirty-four, relatively young and otherwise healthy patients with hypothyroidism who were kept on T_4 and had normal TSH levels. She used several tests—similar to those used in the European studies—to evaluate quality of life, mood, and multiple types of memory. The results surprised Samuels. She did not expect to see that despite having normal TSH levels, T_4-treated patients had consistent decrements in health status, psychological function, working memory, and motor learning compared to euthyroid controls. She published her work in March 2007.[7]

Since then, one more large study has been performed, this time at the University Medical Center Groningen, in the northern Netherlands, and published in February 2017. This study used a series of self-administered questionnaires to study about 360 patients with hypothyroidism treated with T_4. The results were then compared with matched healthy individuals. Again, female patients in Groningen who were using T_4 had lower scores on several domains of health-related quality of life, including physical functioning, vitality, mental health, social functioning, bodily pain, and general health.[8]

*   *   *

Overall, studies published between 2002 and 2007 (and confirmed in 2017) in Europe and the United States show uncontroverted evidence that some T_4-treated patients with normal TSH levels do not feel well and have impaired mood and cognitive functions. Given the prevalence of hypothyroidism, this ends up representing millions of patients. These findings confirm what patients have told us all along about difficulty focusing, memory issues, and sluggishness. They have a difficult time returning to a normal life. My fellow physicians should believe them.

I find it fascinating that physicians in Europe responded much faster to symptomatic patients than in the United States. The British Thyroid Foundation created space for these patients to express their concerns, and this led to studies in Cardiff and Amsterdam. In contrast, the study in Portland, Oregon, only serendipitously touched on the problem (but obtained very similar results). At the time of this book's writing, no other such studies have been completed in the United States. As we saw in chapter 3, this contrast played out in 2012, when both European and American professional societies published guidelines on the treatment of hypothyroidism. Whereas the Europeans recognized that not all patients on T_4 feel well, and spelled out how to approach and treat symptomatic patients, the physicians in the United States merely reaffirmed the efficacy of T_4 to treat hypothyroidism.

*   *   *

One of the complaints that we physicians frequently hear from patients with hypothyroidism on T_4 is difficulty managing body weight. Of course, overweight is so much more frequent these days that many patients might express the same concern, whether they have hypothyroidism or not. However, patients with hypothyroidism on T_4 do seem to have a propensity to gain weight. Sarah Peterson, a clinical nutritionist whom I met at Rush University in Chicago, studied this phenomenon. Peterson looked at data collected from the United States National Health and Nutrition Examination Survey (NHANES) from 2001 to 2012. The strength of the NHANES program lies in the fact that it is a population-based survey designed to collect information on the health and nutrition of the American household. It is not a clinical trial in which participants enroll given their interest in a specific disease. Participants are selected using a random sampling method. The survey examines a nationally representative sample of about five thousand people each year. The interview includes demographic, socioeconomic, dietary, and health-related questions. It also looks at medical, dental, and physiological measurements, as well as laboratory tests administered by highly trained medical personnel. Once the results are processed, they are posted online and are publicly available.

Peterson looked at about ten thousand individuals on T_4 and identified almost five hundred individuals who were treated with T_4 and had normal TSH levels.[9] She also identified the same number of control individuals that matched for sex, age, ethnic background, and TSH levels. She then compared more than fifty NHANES parameters in both groups of individuals. While most parameters did not show differences, individuals on T_4 reported lower physical activity and were found to be about ten pounds heavier, despite consuming fewer calories. They were also 30–40% more likely to be on antidepressants, statins, or beta-blockers. Furthermore, individuals on T_4 were found to have an "increased likelihood to experience confusion/memory problems" and a "decreased likelihood to state excellent or good health conditions" when compared with matched controls.

Besides the cognitive issues, is it possible that despite T_4 treatment, some patients remain slightly hypometabolic? The increase in body weight and statin utilization seems to indicate that yes, they do. But how can we be sure of this? A good first step is to look at metabolic parameters typically sensitive to thyroid hormones. The rate of metabolism is one such parameter. It indicates how many calories a given individual is burning per day. For example, a forty-year-old, 150-pound, 5-foot-6 woman burns approximately 1,400 calories per day, whereas a forty-year-old, 180-pound, 6-foot man burns about 1,800 calories per day. In approximate terms, these individuals should eat about 1,400 and 1,800 calories per day, respectively, to maintain stable body weight. If the rate of metabolism slows down and the food intake remains the same, there will be a tendency to gain weight in both cases. Overt hypothyroid patients have a slower metabolism (burn fewer calories), hence easily feel cold and have a tendency to gain weight. Yes, restoring the metabolic rate to normal should be a paramount goal of the treatment of hypothyroidism.

As I looked into such studies, I saw with surprise that T_4-treated patients with normal TSH levels continue to exhibit slower than normal metabolic rates. Colum Gorman, a clinician-scientist at the Mayo Clinic, obtained in 1979 a hint that this was the case.[10] He measured the metabolic rate of a group of seven patients with hypothyroidism before and during treatment with T_4. While the T_4 tablets normalized TSH levels in all patients, they also accelerated the metabolic rate but failed to normalize it. In five patients, the metabolic rate remained slower than normal. Only in two patients did the metabolic rate return to normal levels.

I was puzzled by those results, and in the summer of 2016, I called Gorman. He said he didn't think much about it at the time, as he expected that eventually the metabolic rate would return to normal in all patients. This sounded very reasonable. However, by the time he studied his patients, they had been on T_4 for six months. I know exactly what Gorman meant, because I felt the same way for almost all my professional life. According to the conferences I attended and the papers I read, there was simply no reason to suspect that T_4 wasn't doing its job.

Then I found another study, this one by Chip Ridgway, who in 1980 was working at Mass General Hospital in Boston.[11] He and his colleagues studied patients with hypothyroidism treated with T_4 and found that once TSH had normalized, the metabolic rate had not.

Thirty-six years later, in 2016, using more sophisticated technology, Mary Samuels, the clinician-scientist in Portland, studied the metabolic rate of eighty women on T_4 with normal TSH levels.[12] Samuels confirmed that these women had a 4% slower metabolic rate when compared with sixteen healthy controls.

The slower metabolic rate in T_4-treated patients has also been observed in Europe, and in patients who are obese.[13] A group of physicians working at the Policlinico Hospital in Monza, Italy, looked at eighty-five obese patients with hypothyroidism on T_4, with normal TSH levels, and compared them with about 650 obese women. The metabolic rate was 6% slower in women on T_4, even when results were adjusted for age, body mass index, body composition, and level of physical activity.

This is a big deal, with certain consequences to the overall metabolism. The reduction in metabolic rate detected in the T_4-treated patients may seem small; with time, though, it is bound to have consequences. Imagine a car going at 50 mph and another car at a slightly slower speed, at 48 mph. This might seem a small difference, but, at the end of twenty-four hours, the two cars will be almost fifty miles apart. Thus, maintaining a 4–6% lower metabolic rate for months or years will have a major impact on the overall metabolism.

I cannot think of anything more relevant for patients with hypothyroidism than this. And I can't understand why more emphasis has not been given to these findings. These studies, across decades, show that treatment with T_4 does not fully restore metabolic rate.

My patients with hypothyroidism have been complaining forever that the disease makes them gain weight, and I kept telling them it is not true. Repeatedly I told them that restoring TSH levels is sufficient to normalize metabolism. It was what I had been taught, and I was wrong.

*　*　*

Sometimes, research conducted on laboratory animals can carry significant clinical implications. In 2015, while I was trying to understand what was happening with my two patients in Miami, I cast a wide net to identify systems that remain abnormal during treatment with T_4.[14] I asked my students to look at approximately one thousand rats with hypothyroidism that had been placed on T_4 therapy. A large number was needed to detect small differences. Once TSH levels had been normalized, we studied multiple organs.

I was surprised to see clear signs of hypothyroidism in the liver, skeletal muscle, and different areas of the brain, despite normalization of TSH levels with T_4. The elevated levels of cholesterol in the circulation stood out among the findings. It was unexpected. Yes, cholesterol levels are affected by thyroid hormones. Overt hypothyroid patients have high cholesterol levels. But treatment with T_4—to normal TSH levels—should have restored cholesterol levels to normal as well. It didn't. Levels were lowered as compared to overt hypothyroid rats, but not to the normal reference range. What fascinated me was that rats placed on combination therapy ($T_4 + T_3$) exhibited normal cholesterol levels.

I did not immediately follow up on these findings. However, they did not go unnoticed in Japan. Two years later, a group of physicians at Kuma Hospital in Kobe, Japan, reported the assessment of about thirty patients who had their cholesterol checked before and one year after surgical removal of the thyroid gland and treatment with T_4. Just like the rats with hypothyroidism, patients on T_4 exhibited higher cholesterol levels in the blood despite normal TSH levels. In 2019, physicians in Korea did a similar study, this time with more than a thousand women. The study also revealed elevation of cholesterol levels two years after thyroid surgery and treatment with T_4.[15]

While she was a fellow in my laboratory, Elizabeth McAninch identified sixty-five studies that compared almost two thousand patients treated with T_4 with more than fourteen thousand healthy controls. McAninch and colleagues concluded that cholesterol levels remained elevated despite the normalization of plasma TSH levels.[16] The results of these studies were consistent, but the magnitude of the elevation in cholesterol was small. I expected more based on the study we did on rats. Then I remembered that Sarah Peterson and her colleagues had found that patients on T_4 are more likely to be taking cholesterol-lowering medicines (statins).[17] This could potentially be minimizing an otherwise substantial elevation in cholesterol levels.

My next move was to ask Thayer Idrees, a clinical fellow in my group, to follow up on Peterson's findings and study the utilization of statins in patients taking T_4. He looked at approximately eleven thousand patients up to three years before and three years after they were placed on T_4.[18] What he saw was noteworthy. In this cohort, the number of patients on a statin medication increased from about 20% to 25% *after* they were placed on T_4, and for those who were already on a statin, the strength of the medication increased by about 30%. Most patients were placed on a statin one to two years after they started on T_4, at a time when they had normal TSH levels. This is a strong indication that treatment with T_4 does not fully normalize the levels of cholesterol. While we do not understand why that is, these findings fit nicely with the idea that the liver remains slightly hypothyroid despite treatment with T_4. This is what one would expect when T_3 levels are below normal range.

I wanted to confirm these results in a different setting. I called Rui Maciel, the physician-scientist and my former mentor in São Paulo. Maciel is associated with one of the largest clinical laboratories in Brazil, and—at his insistence—every patient who comes for a clinical visit is briefly interviewed and asked about their list of medications. With the help of his team of computer analysts, we looked at approximately five and a half million interviews collected over ten years and saw that in both sexes and at every age range, taking T_4 increases the odds of being on statin medication by about twofold.

Then I spoke to another colleague, Fernando Fernandes, the medical director for a large pharmaceutical company in São Paulo. With help of his team, we also looked at prescription patterns by primary care physicians in Brazil. We wanted to test the hypothesis that when a patient is placed on T_4, sooner or later the physician will also place that patient on statin medications. This is feasible only because T_4 is exclusively used to treat patients with hypothyroidism, and T_3 or thyroid extracts are not commercially available in Brazil. After analyzing approximately one hundred million prescriptions written during 2018, we saw that the 1.4 million patients on T_4 were about one and a half times more likely to also have received a prescription of statin when compared to controls (patients not receiving T_4, and matched for age and sex).

*   *   *

The slower metabolic rate and elevated cholesterol levels in patients with hypothyroidism treated with T_4 suggest that these patients show a residual metabolic dysregulation despite normalization of TSH. This is in addition to the cognitive impairment and lower quality of life exhibited by millions of patients. Although these findings do not allow us to conclude that thyroid-hormone action is impaired in T_4-treated patients, when taken together, they paint a very suggestive picture that this is in fact the case.

We definitively need to improve the treatment of hypothyroidism. The idea that treatment for hypothyroidism is simple, case closed, is gone. The case is being reopened across the globe, and new information is obtained daily. This is a sad story. Patients' suffering was predictable based on what we knew during the 1970s. We physicians should have understood the possibility that something was wrong and tested for this clinically. I am disappointed in myself for not realizing this issue sooner.

*　*　*

If my medical colleagues reading this book take away just one message, it would be that the fact that the majority of patients are doing well does not necessarily mean that the symptoms experienced by the minority are not real or are not thyroid related. It just means that we physicians need to do a better job of understanding how to treat hypothyroidism.

How can this be fixed, is the pressing question before us. To fix it, we first need to understand it, to understand the underlying mechanisms that cause the symptoms to linger. This is what is discussed in the next three chapters. I continue to thread my own story with the ongoing breakthroughs of recent decades against the historical breakthroughs of an earlier era. I challenge dogma and the modern treatment of hypothyroidism—we need to go beyond TSH testing for adjusting the dose of T_4.

CHAPTER 10
TSH Isn't a Magic Bullet

Measuring the circulating levels of TSH—the hormone that stimulates the thyroid gland to function—is a phenomenal tool to diagnose hypothyroidism. It became the gold standard adopted worldwide because of two facts: (1) Most of what the thyroid does is secrete T_4; and (2) TSH secretion responds rapidly to minimal changes in T_4 levels. Thus, monitoring TSH levels in the circulation to assess thyroid function makes sense.

The mechanisms explaining the exquisite TSH sensitivity of T_4 were defined by Enrique Silva and Reed Larsen, both of whom I had the privilege of working with and learning from, for many years. In the early 1970s, they did not know each other, but they were both curious about observations they made independently, Silva in Santiago, Chile, and Larsen in Boston. They found that iodine deficiency produces a drastic drop in T_4 (but not T_3), and yet no signs (or symptoms) of hypothyroidism could be detected in rats (or humans) with this condition. They wondered how T_4 could be so important for TSH regulation and yet, its drop in circulation did not cause signs or symptoms of hypothyroidism.[1]

Later, when working together at the Brigham and Women's Hospital in Boston, they were inspired by Jack Oppenheimer's recent discovery that organs respond to T_3 but much less to T_4. They predicted a mechanism inside the various organs (deiodination, which is the removal of an iodine atom from T_4) that activates the actions of T_4. In other words, they considered that even with low T_4 levels, a deiodinase could amplify the effects of T_4 (by converting it to T_3).

But they were not sure how to proceed, how to test their idea. At that time, both Silva and Larsen were not known in the deiodinase field, and there was only one known deiodinase (D1), which they suspected was not involved.

Larsen went to Silva's office to strategize. (His office was unusual, a wedge-shaped space behind an elevator shaft.) They discussed different possibilities and decided to do a test trial, first looking at the effects of T_3 on TSH secretion. As planned, a few days later, Silva injected rats with radioactive T_3 and saw a drop in circulating TSH at the same time that radioactive T_3 was building up in the pituitary gland. This meant that T_3 inhibits TSH through its actions in the pituitary gland. Part 1 of their plan was accomplished.

They continued with the strategy crafted in Silva's office and moved to the second part of their plan: to test the hypothesis that the pituitary gland takes up T_4 and converts it to T_3, and that this could be the amplification mechanism they were looking for. But the technical details of the plan were still not clear.

Here is when fate took care of things by putting Silva and Larsen together. Their skills complemented each other's. Silva has an analytical mind, capable of planning experiments and rapidly identifying and solving problems. Larsen has the ability to put things into perspective, always looking at the big picture when interpreting the results. In retrospect, few investigators at that time could have addressed this question so elegantly.

To test their hypothesis, Silva and Larsen next injected rats with radioactive T_4 and looked for radioactive T_3 in the pituitary gland. But the rat's pituitary gland is a very tiny organ. To detect anything, they had to inject large amounts of T_4, which made the experiment too expensive. To save money, they decided to make radioactive T_4 themselves. They had a special room in the basement of the old Peter Bent Brigham Hospital in Boston, accessed through a long, dark, and narrow staircase. (I used that room a few times to make my own T_4.) The room was poorly illuminated and was shielded with two-inch lead bricks to block the radioactivity. In this room, they carefully mixed T_3 and radioactive iodine, keeping it behind the bricks for thirty seconds, sufficient time for the radioactive iodine to be incorporated into T_3, producing radioactive T_4.

Unfortunately, despite injecting a lot of radioactive T_4 in the rats, the amount of radioactive T_3 produced in the pituitary was still very small and hard to detect. Thankfully, Larsen had an idea. For some time, he had been keeping rabbits in the basement and garage of his house in Brookline, to develop anti-T_3 antibodies (these bind to T_3 and don't easily let go)—his goal was to develop good antibodies to measure T_3 in the circulation. Larsen had his kids, then very young, to tend the rabbits. The antibodies he developed were so good that they were used for decades, including in many of Silva's and my studies.

Reed Larsen asked his fellow at the time, Motomori Izumi, to attach the anti-T_3 antibodies to microscopic beads (called Sepharose), which were later used to trap and concentrate the radioactive T_3, separating it from radioactive T_4. The strategy worked. By using the anti-T_3 beads Silva trapped the radioactive T_3. He and Larsen saw that a few hours after the rats were injected with radioactive T_4, TSH in the circulation fell and, at the same time, radioactive T_3 built up in the pituitary gland, nailing down the mechanism. They had discovered that T_4 is converted to T_3 inside the pituitary gland, and that is why T_4 can be so important in the mechanism that regulates TSH secretion.

Only years later did scientists figure out that D2 was the enzyme converting T_4 to T_3 in the pituitary gland, at the center of the mechanism that controls TSH regulation.

These studies were done in rats, but they revealed such novel aspects of thyroid-hormone action that they radically changed the way people thought about the regulation of TSH secretion, including in humans.[2] Although some aspects of these mechanisms remained unclear at the time, and would only be elucidated much later, the profound impact of those studies rapidly found its way into clinical practice. They constitute the mechanistic basis for the clinical paradigm in use today that hypothyroidism can be diagnosed by looking at T_4 and TSH levels in the circulation.

* * *

Around the same time, in 1975, Jerome (Jerry) Hershman, a physician-scientist at the West Los Angeles VA hospital, was also studying the mechanisms regulating TSH secretion. His studies were in humans. Thinking along the same lines as Silva and Larsen did, Hershman wanted to inhibit T_4-to-T_3 conversion and see if that affected TSH secretion. The only way of doing this at the time was to treat volunteers with a drug that can inhibit T_4-to-T_3 conversion. In the 1970s, D1 was the only deiodinase known, and propylthiouracil was known as a potent D1 inhibitor. Hershman hypothesized that inhibiting D1 would markedly elevate TSH levels, equivalent to a drop in T_4 levels.

To test his hypothesis, Hershman and two of his fellows, David Geffner and Mizuo Azukizawa, recruited individuals with hypothyroidism who were being treated with T_4 and maintained a normal TSH. His patients were admitted and received a large dose of the D1 inhibitor (propylthiouracil) for several days. Treatment with the inhibitor caused a progressive drop in T_3 levels in the circulation. But the drop was modest, only about 20% at the end of the experiment, without changes in T_4 levels. The drop in T_3, albeit small, did elevate TSH levels in the circulation.[3] Together with Silva and Larsen's results, this study indicated that, in addition to T_4, the pituitary gland is also constantly monitoring circulating-T_3 levels.

What Hershman did not know was that he had obtained the first evidence of the importance of the D2 pathway in humans. He showed that in T_4-treated patients, most (80%) of the T_3 in the circulation is produced by the D2 pathway (which is insensitive to propylthiouracil). D1 does play a small role (20%), but it is clear that the D2 pathway is key for producing most T_3 in the circulation of T_4-treated patients.

I always show a slide of these seminal studies in my lectures. And so I did several years ago when my friend Jorge Mestman invited me to lecture at USC in Los Angeles. The next day, Mestman took me to a meeting of the Los Angeles Thyroid Club, where I lectured again. I showed my slide with Hershman's results. He was in the audience, and at the end, he humbly said, "Tony, I am always surprised that you still show these old studies from 1975 in your lectures, and today I am going to surprise you by introducing you to David Geffner"—his former fellow who did the studies and was also in the audience. I was so happy to have met him. I congratulated and thanked them for their studies and said that from then on, I was going to refer to the studies as Geffner and Hershman's studies.

*　*　*

Thanks to Silva and Larsen's and Geffner and Hershman's studies, we now know that the D2 pathway is at the center of TSH regulation and the production of T_3 for circulation. In other words, the success or failure of T_4 as a treatment for hypothyroidism depends greatly on D2.

By treating patients with hypothyroidism with T_4, we are counting on the D2 pathway to normalize TSH secretion—given that T_4 is converted to T_3 in the pituitary gland via D2. We are also counting on the D2 pathway to provide T_3 for the circulation—given that T_4 is converted to T_3 in many other organs via D2. So, by choosing T_4 as the standard treatment for hypothyroidism, without knowing at the time, physicians placed the D2 pathway at the center of the therapy. They relied heavily on the D2 pathway to produce the right amounts of T_3 at the right place and at the right time. And of course, any changes or defects in the D2 pathway will negatively impact the effectiveness of treatment with T_4.

*   *   *

Studies in Reed Larsen's laboratory first discovered the D2 pathway, and over the years he focused on everything about it. One of the things he was curious about was why D2 is short lived. Don St. Germain, the physician-scientist at Dartmouth, discovered that in a regular cell, D2 is destroyed so fast that, every fifty minutes, half of all D2 is gone and more needs to be made.[4] He also discovered that every time D2 converts T_4 to T_3, it ends up being destroyed.[5] Yes, it is what I call self-destructive or suicidal behavior; D2 pays with its own life the price for converting T_4 to T_3. As a consequence, when there is little T_4 around, as in hypothyroidism, D2 accumulates everywhere, producing T_3 from any tiny bit of T_4. In contrast, when there is an excess of T_4, D2 disappears, nowhere to be found, limiting the amount of T_3 that can be produced from T_4 at any given time.

How is it that D2 is destroyed so fast and its destruction is accelerated by T_4? Around 1996, Larsen was trying to answer that question, but nothing he tested helped. Then Jack Leonard, the scientist at the University of Massachusetts in Worcester, published a study showing that the short D2 lifespan depended on cellular energy.[6] This meant that cells had to use their energy storage to destroy D2.

Larsen rapidly seized on Leonard's finding, as he remembered that the skeletal muscle also uses energy to destroy its proteins through a system called the proteasome. Proteasomes are large protein complexes within cells that function as a vacuum cleaner, moving around and disassembling proteins. Larsen knew about this because his friend from across Longwood Avenue, Alfred Goldberg, a world expert on this system, had developed a new drug that inhibited the proteasomes. Larsen wasted no time, and had his fellow Jaime Steinsapir use this inhibitor. Sure enough, the inhibitor preserved D2's life, unequivocally showing that this system is involved.[7]

The ability of this pathway to destroy proteins is so developed that cells carefully control when and where to unleash its power. In the case of D2, Balázs Gereben and I later showed that this system destroys only those D2 molecules that have been earmarked (tagged) for destruction—tagging, in this case, means attachment to a much smaller protein known as ubiquitin.[8] Once tagged, D2 becomes a target and is destroyed. Gereben, a scientist at the Institute of Experimental Medicine in Budapest, Hungary, is a phenomenal molecular biologist, exceptionally gifted when it comes to manipulating DNA molecules. Even though he is in Budapest, we became good friends and published dozens of studies together. In 2021 we received an NIH grant to study the effects of D2 tagging in the brain.

I became very interested in understanding more about how D2 is tagged. One of the things that had been in the back of my mind was the observation by Isabelle Callebaut, the French scientist with whom I collaborated to unveil the molecular structure of the deiodinases, that D2 has a unique short loop made up of eighteen amino acids, not present in the other deiodinases.[9] I was fortunate that, at that time, Monica Dentice, a postdoc from the University of Naples in Italy, had just arrived for a fellowship in my laboratory in Boston. So, Dentice and I investigated this loop and discovered that the loop is the key for D2's tagging. As it turned out, several scavenger proteins are constantly hunting down D2. They identify D2 by its unique loop, which becomes more visible to the scavengers at the moment D2 converts T_4 to T_3. When it happens, the scavengers recognize D2 and rapidly tag it for destruction. Once the tag is in place, it is the end for D2.[10]

Why such an elaborate mechanism to regulate D2? This is the way our bodies have found to prevent too much conversion of T_4 to T_3. Recall that T_3 is a very potent molecule. Hence, the body developed safeguards against its excessive production. Relatively speaking, the more T_4 is available, the less T_3 will be produced because, at every round of T_4-to-T_3 conversion, more D2 is tagged and destroyed.

But there is another twist to the story. More or less at the same time, Cynthia Curcio, a graduate student in my lab, made the remarkable discovery that D2 tagging could be reversible! Indeed, tagged D2 can be untagged and rescued from destruction. Working with yeast that had been engineered to express D2, Curcio discovered two proteins that bind tagged D2 and untag it, protecting D2 from destruction.[11]

These findings were a big deal. We learned that the conversion of T_4 to T_3 via D2 is regulated by the sheer amount of T_4 around the cell. Tagging D2 sends it for destruction and slows down T_3 production. In contrast, untagging D2 rescues it from destruction and reactivates T_3 production.

*　*　*

Only with time, I realized the clinical implications of these findings. Think about this question: With all these elaborate mechanisms to modify D2 activity, is it possible that D2 regulation is not the same in all organs? In other words, is it possible that the balance between the tagging and untagging of D2 is different from organ to organ? This is such an important question, one that holds the key to the failures of treatment for hypothyroidism with T_4.

Subsequent studies in my laboratory have shown that the tagging of D2 in the structures involved in TSH secretion is a seemingly *inefficient* process.[12] In other words, T_4 is converted to T_3 without causing much tagging of D2. There is some D2 tagging, but there is also massive untagging of D2, rescuing it from destruction. As a consequence, D2 accumulates in the pituitary gland and activates T_4 to T_3 very efficiently, lowering TSH secretion.

In contrast, in other organs, where D2 supplies T_3 to the circulation, D2 tagging is very *efficient* and there is minimal untagging going on. That means that as you are taking T_4 tablets and the T_4 levels increase, D2 is immediately tagged and destroyed, limiting the conversion of T_4-to-T_3. As a consequence, less T_3 is produced for the circulation and the rest of the body. That certainly is a factor in the residual metabolic symptoms—slower metabolic rate, difficulty losing weight, higher cholesterol levels—observed in some of the T_4-treated patients with hypothyroidism.

This scenario sets the stage for a disconnect between TSH and T_3 levels. If this is correct, a regimen of T_4 may normalize TSH levels while T_3 levels remain low. Indeed, as we will see in chapter 11, it is not practical to simultaneously normalize T_3 and TSH levels in the circulation when using T_4 to treat patients with hypothyroidism.

It took me years to figure out the complete mechanism involved. It started in 2007 at a conference in a cold, snowy Colorado. Balázs Gereben was mapping where in the brain the untagging machinery could be found. I wanted to present the data in my talk at the symposium, so I was downloading the brain pictures as fast as he was sending them. I was in awe when I saw that the brain area that controls TSH secretion is one of the few areas that contain the D2 untagging machinery.[13] What followed was a frantic search for additional pieces of the puzzle, which culminated in Chicago in 2015.[14]

In practical terms, I believe this is how the unbalance occurs in patients with hypothyroidism. Let us consider my hypothyroid patient Olivia, back when she was first placed on T_4. As she started the treatment, her T_4 levels were low and her TSH levels were high. The daily T_4 tablets increased her level of T_4, which was converted to T_3 in the pituitary gland (by D2), thereby reducing the TSH levels. As D2 was tagged in the pituitary (due to T_4-to-T_3 conversion), it was also rapidly untagged, and the local production of T_3 via D2 remained steadily high.

At the same time, something different was happening in the organs that have D2 and produce T_3 for the circulation and the rest of the body. The rise in T_4 levels was followed by a rise in T_3 levels due to the conversion of T_4 to T_3 by D2. But the increase in T_3 levels occurred at a much slower pace because D2 was being flagged for destruction and not much untagging was going on. As a result, the amount of T_3 produced for the circulation was progressively less.

Therefore, inhibiting TSH secretion with T_4 is a very efficient process—D2 in the pituitary gland and hypothalamus continuously produces T_3 without much tagging. In contrast, T_4-to-T_3 conversion in other organs is not as efficient—while the T_4 levels in the circulation increase, D2 is lost to tagging and destruction, and T_3 levels lag.

Thus, because of the differences in D2 tagging, it is conceivable that in patients treated with T_4, TSH levels reach the normal reference range at a dose of T_4 that is not sufficient to fully normalize circulating-T_3 levels. If this is correct—and I believe it is—the disconnect in D2 tagging explains why measuring TSH levels is a phenomenal tool to diagnose hypothyroidism, but it is not nearly as good to assess the effectiveness of treatment *if only* T_4 *is being administered.*

*   *   *

TSH levels should be interpreted with caution when assessing therapy for hypothyroidism. In the next chapter, we will explore the current understanding of the crucial importance of T_3 levels, which goes a long way toward explaining the divergence between traditional treatments and contemporary treatment with T_4 only.

A major step here will be to focus on T_3 levels and get you familiarized with the idea that for healthy individuals, preserving T_3 levels is very important. This is a new concept that evolved in recent years in part from studies done in my laboratory. In the absence of a healthy thyroid, preserving T_3 levels is challenging, which has consequences for the treatment of hypothyroidism. I find this to be a critical point given that physicians do not consider T_3 levels as an important factor in the treatment of hypothyroidism.

CHAPTER 11

Missing Clues and T_3

Enrique Silva always talked about Jack Oppenheimer. To put it simply, Oppenheimer was a god for many of us in the field. Born in Egelsbach, Germany, Oppenheimer emigrated to New Jersey at age ten and became one of the most influential thyroidologists of his time. His knowledge of mathematics, chemistry, and physiology made him a leader in the field of thyroid-hormone metabolism and action. Oppenheimer pioneered many breakthroughs in endocrinology, including the discovery that cells respond predominantly to T_3, not to T_4.

He made people nervous when in conferences he stood up, went to the microphone, and asked pointed questions. During the week before my first presentation at the American Thyroid Association annual meeting in 1986, I rehearsed the slides with Silva as he played Oppenheimer's role, asking tough questions. When I finally gave my talk, Oppenheimer was of course the first to ask a question. (And despite my preparation, I was so nervous that I completely misunderstood what he was asking.)

Jack Oppenheimer was also a skilled clinician working out of Montefiore Medical Center and Albert Einstein College of Medicine in the Bronx. He published in 1974 in the *New England Journal of Medicine* one of the first studies in which about forty-five patients with hypothyroidism were treated with T_4.[1] Even from this early study, it was clear that patients exhibited lower T_3 levels in the circulation. This was potentially a major red flag because Oppenheimer himself discovered that T_3 is the active thyroid hormone that resolves symptoms of hypothyroidism.

The fact that Oppenheimer's group reported this finding, in my mind, makes it all the more surprising that it didn't have any impact on treatment. I spoke to Martin Surks in the spring of 2021, a physician-scientist at Montefiore Medical Center in New York, one of the authors of the study, and asked him if they were surprised with the lower T_3 levels. He said the main focus of the study was to understand how synthetic T_4 is metabolized and distributed through the body. He did not remember any specific discussions around T_3 levels, which leads me to conclude that they were so excited with there being so much T_3 in the circulation of T_4-treated patients that a minor difference (about 10% lower) did not catch their attention as being clinically relevant.

Oppenheimer's was not the only study showing lower T_3 levels. Clark Sawin and Jerry Hershman, respectively at the Boston and West Los Angeles VA hospitals, and colleagues compared T_4 with the low-tech old treatment, thyroid extract, in fifteen patients with hypothyroidism. They concluded in 1978 that T_4 and thyroid extract were "equivalent"—both could effectively normalize TSH levels and resolve obvious signs and symptoms of overt hypothyroidism (at that time, residual symptoms had not yet been formally recognized, so their presence in these patients was not studied). Nonetheless, they did note that patients on T_4 had slightly lower circulating-T_3 levels.[2] In 1982, it was Lew Braverman and Sidney Ingbar's turn, both at the Beth Israel Hospital in Boston, to find lower circulating-T_3 levels in patients taking Synthroid.[3]

The findings of lower T_3 levels in patients receiving T_4 were clear. By any standard, thyroid experts and physicians in general should have been alarmed, especially considering the reports (anecdotal at the time) that patients placed on T_4 or switched to T_4 from thyroid extract remained symptomatic. But they didn't. These dots were not connected, and no appropriately designed effectiveness and safety trials were ever conducted. The thyroid community embraced T_4 adjusted by TSH levels and moved fast toward making it and defending it as the standard of care to treat hypothyroidism.

General acceptance that T_3 levels are lower in T_4-treated patients, and the potential downstream consequences, have not been straightforward. I have lectured at conferences about lower T_3 levels in T_4-treated patients, but many of my colleagues remain skeptical. I have been told that "Jack Oppenheimer must be rolling in his grave," or that I "have been selective and biased on the data [I] presented," and that "rats are not humans." These criticisms made me doubt myself. Is it possible that I misread Oppenheimer's study? Have I misunderstood the data? That is the worst nightmare for a scientist. Once, when I was in a hotel for a conference, I ran upstairs to my room after such criticism and looked at Oppenheimer's paper on my computer one more time. No, I was right: T_3 levels were indeed reported lower in the group of T_4-treated patients.

∗ ∗ ∗

In the early 1950s, Jack Gross and Rosalind Pitt-Rivers identified T_3 in the blood and found it to be about three times more potent than T_4.[4] This led them to speculate that T_3 was the active form of thyroid hormone.

T_3 circulates in the blood, but two-thirds of its content in the body is located inside the organs, where it exerts its effects. However, T_3 is not a stationary hormone. It is in constant flux between circulating blood and the organs. T_3 levels in the circulation as measured in blood should give an idea of how much T_3

is in the organs, accelerating metabolism, lowering cholesterol levels, and performing its other important functions. The only exception is the brain. In the brain, most T_3 is produced locally via D2; thus, T_3 levels in the circulation do not reflect the content of T_3 in the brain.

Nonetheless, the detection of T_3 levels in the circulation has not been used clinically in the *diagnosis* of hypothyroidism. There are a few reasons for that.

- Eighty percent of what the thyroid produces is T_4, not T_3. Most T_3 in the blood is produced outside the thyroid gland, through the deiodinases that converts T_4 to T_3. Thus, to find out whether the thyroid gland is failing, it makes more sense to measure T_4 levels in the circulation, and not T_3.
- The body adjusts T_3 production to defend T_3 levels. A primary directive is to keep T_3 levels within normal range. In other words, the brain areas that control the thyroid adjust themselves and tolerate abnormal levels of TSH and T_4, so that T_3 levels are maintained within normal range. As a result, a drop in T_3 is probably one of the last things that happen as the thyroid becomes progressively less active. So, measuring T_3 levels would not provide an early diagnosis of hypothyroidism.
- TSH levels are exquisitely sensitive to even minimal variations of circulating-T_4 levels, rapidly climbing above normal range in response to a fall in T_4.

Therefore, the diagnosis of hypothyroidism is traditionally made through the combination of low T_4 and elevated TSH levels. Circulating-T_3 levels have no part in it.

* * *

Now, here is a tricky question. Should we also dismiss circulating-T_3 levels in the *management* of patients with hypothyroidism? If you've been following my argument, you'll know my answer now is an obvious no—but there is no consensus, and I can't explain why. I can't understand why the primary goal of treatment of hypothyroidism isn't the normalization of T_3 levels. Instead, the primary goal is to normalize TSH levels. T_3 levels in the blood have been left out of this equation. It is assumed that if you normalize TSH, you will eventually normalize T_3 as well. But we know this is not true.

If guidelines were to include T_3 levels in the management of hypothyroidism, then physicians would need to face the reality that T_3 levels are frequently in the lower limit of normal, and many times, below normal. This would need to be explained and discussed with patients. A patient could easily say: If my T_3 levels are below normal, why not add T_3 to my treatment plan? Physicians are not prepared to face this question simply because we have not been trained to consider T_3 in hypothyroidism.

Finding lower-than-normal T_3 levels would prompt physicians to do something about it, right? But what? If we increase the dose of T_4, we might risk suppressing TSH levels, and there is no guarantee that this will normalize T_3 levels. Alternatively, we could prescribe T_3. However, guidelines are historically against the use of T_3 to normalize T_3 levels.

Patients ask about these points all the time, and I do not have a reasonable answer other than agreeing with them. This is such an important point, but current guidelines simply do not mention it. Very few people in the academic world talk about this.

*　*　*

Once Val Galton at Dartmouth identified and cloned the D2 gene,[5] she worked quickly with Mark Schneider, a scientist in her laboratory, to inactivate the gene in mice. They created a mouse in which the D2 gene had been inactivated—knocked out.[6] This allowed them to figure out what happens when the D2 pathway is defective. During the 2000 International Thyroid Congress in Kyoto, I was delighted to hear Schneider present on the successful creation of such a mouse. After we returned to Boston, Larsen called Galton and asked for a pair of breeding couples, so that we too could study those mice in Boston.

Galton graciously agreed to share her mice; soon after that, Reed Larsen and I drove from Boston to Dartmouth to pick them up. On our way there, we talked about a bunch of things, including potential experiments we could do with these new mice. He wanted the mice for studies of TSH regulation and I to study brown adipose tissue, the organ that produces heat and maintains body temperature in small rodents.

The drive was just a couple of hours. The Dartmouth-Hitchcock medical center was fantastic, a series of modern buildings surrounded by what seemed dense forest. The group showed us their laboratories and we had lunch. That is when Don St. Germain came up with a really interesting idea: What if we crossed the D2 knockout mouse with a mouse that had a severe defect in D1, the other deiodinase that converts T_4 to T_3. Larsen had studied the D1-deficient mouse years before, and so St. Germain thought it appropriate for us to do these studies. We did not discuss it further, but I assumed all of us in the room expected the resulting mouse, with a combined defect in D1 and D2, to have low T_3 levels in the circulation. We drove back to Boston excited with the experiments each of us had planned.

Once in Boston, Lucia de Jesus, a graduate student from São Paulo, started the brown adipose tissue studies. I also asked another graduate student, Marcelo Christoffolete, to breed the D1-and-D2-deficient mice as St. Germain had suggested. Much to everyone's surprise—and disappointment—the resulting mouse had normal T_3 levels in the circulation![7] How could this be possible without the D1 and D2 pathways? We measured and remeasured, but the results held. I was hoping for a marked drop in circulating T_3, which would have indicated that the deiodinases were very important to sustain T_3 levels. Everybody was. Since T_3 did not drop, I did not think too much about it anymore. As I always say, research is 90% failure and 10% success. We learn from our failures and live off the successes. But Christoffolete had soon to present his doctoral thesis and we had to start putting things together, which forced us to complete the studies and to think.

Others in the lab were also wondering why we continued with this line of work. Why did we want to publish negative results? I did not have an answer then, other than Christoffolete's doctoral thesis and something in my mind that was telling me to continue.

Years later, I realized how important those findings were. Even though we hailed the deiodinases as such important enzymes, we were looking at the fact that in their absence, circulating-T_3 levels were unaffected, remained stable within normal range. The only other source of T_3 in that mouse was the thyroid gland. The results indicated that in the total absence of T_4-to-T_3 conversion, the thyroid gland adjusted itself and increased T_3 production to preserve T_3 levels in the circulation. This was such a surprise to me. I was used to thinking that the thyroid adjusted to circulating-T_4 levels. In the back of my mind, I knew T_3 also played a role, but I would never have thought that the thyroid system adjusts itself based on T_3 levels in the circulation. It makes sense, though. T_3 is the active thyroid hormone.

*   *   *

In retrospect, we should have known that preserving T_3 levels is a priority for the thyroid system. This hierarchy evolved over millions of years in response to biological pressures from the environment, the main one being iodine deficiency. Iodine deficiency shaped the evolution of the thyroid system, and preserving T_3

levels was the best way out. When humans (or rats) experience a shortage of iodine in the food supply, the thyroid gland responds promptly by increasing the relative secretion of T_3—maintaining blood levels of T_3—the active thyroid hormone.

This is showcased in areas of the world where iodine deficiency is still a problem. Inhabitants of these areas frequently exhibit an enlarged thyroid—a goiter—that by sheer size increases the ability to take up iodine and sustain thyroid-hormone production. At the same time, the thyroid reduces its relative production of T_4 and increases the production of T_3, all to preserve the levels of T_3 in the circulation. In turn, lower levels of T_4 accelerate T_4-to-T_3 conversion via D2, contributing to the safeguarding of T_3 levels. Thus, the message is clear: the body is naturally hardwired to defend and preserve circulating-T_3 levels.

But things are very different during the treatment of hypothyroidism with T_4, which causes a slight elevation of T_4 level in the circulation. It is artificial to replace the thyroid secretion, which contains T_4 and T_3, exclusively with T_4. The adaptive mechanisms that evolved over hundreds of millions of years—vertebrates—to function with lower T_4 levels are not able to cope with higher T_4 levels. As a result, normalization of TSH levels with only T_4 is not physiological. It results in T_3 levels that are slightly reduced.

I can't think of anything in nature that causes an elevation in T_4 levels and, as a result, the thyroid and the system that converts T_4 to T_3 did not evolve to handle it adequately. As we will see in the next chapter, it is naive—romantic, even—to think that a system that evolved over millions of years to respond by lowering T_4 levels (caused by iodine deficiency) could function properly when we forcefully raise T_4 levels by treating patients with T_4 only. No wonder T_3 homeostasis is disrupted and its levels in the circulation are relatively lower, in many cases below the normal reference range.

*   *   *

The clinical implications of these observations are dramatic; they cannot be overstated. If preserving T_3 levels is such an imperative mandate, then why are we not monitoring T_3 levels in T_4-treated patients? Why are we not considering T_3 levels when planning the treatment of hypothyroidism?

That thought prompted me to go back and look for more studies that addressed that question. I was trying to figure out whether the deiodinases were prepared to readjust themselves and defend circulating-T_3 levels in the absence of a healthy thyroid gland. The questions were simple: Do T_4-treated patients with normal TSH levels also have normal T_3 levels? Can the deiodinases manage to accelerate T_3 production and defend T_3 levels in the circulation in the absence of a functional thyroid gland?

At first, this seemed like a question with an obvious answer, as most physicians would say: yes, the deiodinases can adjust their function to produce just the right amounts of T_3. I remember vividly lecturing for years and saying exactly that (I still have the slide I used to show). However, as I dug deeper, I saw that this was not the case at all.

Following those three initial studies showing that T_3 levels were not normalized in T_4-treated patients,[8] six other studies involving up to a hundred T_4-treated patients each, found T_3 levels to be relatively lower;[9] although five similar studies were not able to detect differences in T_3 levels.[10] In summary, while all studies agreed that treatment with T_4 can be used to normalize TSH levels, there was great inconsistency around circulating-T_3 levels.

Among the possible explanations for this inconsistency was the relatively small number of patients enrolled in the studies and the great variability of the methods used to measure T_3 levels in the blood. In addition, circulating T_3 is greatly affected by food intake and is usually reduced in patients trying to lose weight by dieting. Thus, it seems that the conclusions of the studies discussed above were blurred by multiple covariates and the involvement of a relatively small number of patients.

*   *   *

Two subsequent studies involving a large number of patients point unequivocally to plasma T_3 being lower in T_4-treated patients.

The first study was serendipitous. Damiano Gullo, a physician at the Garibaldi-Nesima Hospital in Catania, Italy, was curious whether the efficacy of T_4 varies according to the seasons of the year. He runs a busy clinic, so he had complete data sets from about 1,800 T_4-treated thyroidectomized patients. As he and his colleague Adele Latina dug into the numbers and looked for a relationship between TSH levels and the seasons, they were surprised by something else, which they did not expect. They saw that patients treated with T_4 have 17% lower T_3 levels and 12.5% higher T_4 levels in the blood when compared to 3,900 control individuals not taking T_4. It's important to note that all patients had normal TSH levels.[11]

In addition, they observed that about 15% of the T_4-treated patients had abnormally low blood T_3 levels—below the normal reference range! I discussed these results with Gullo in September 2011, during a meeting of the European Thyroid Association in Krakow.

Sarah Peterson and her colleagues did the second study using NHANES data (2001–2012).[12] As we saw, combing through this database, Peterson identified about 470 individuals taking T_4. The researchers then identified an additional 470 individuals of the same sex, age, ethnic background, with the same TSH level. The idea was to obtain two very similar populations that differed in only one key area—treatment with T$_4$. Lo and behold, individuals taking T$_4$ had about 10% lower circulating-T$_3$ levels as compared to the matched controls.

These two studies were very significant given the large number of patients involved and the fact that they employed matched controls, including matching for TSH values. Unequivocally, we now know that treatment of patients with hypothyroidism with T$_4$ that normalizes TSH levels does not necessarily restore T$_3$ levels in the body.

* * *

The brain, the pituitary gland, and the thyroid gland are hardwired to defend and preserve T$_3$ levels. Thus, finding that T$_4$-treated patients have about 10–15% lower T$_3$ levels was a big deal.

Why? Recall that circulating-T$_3$ levels reflect the amount of T$_3$ in most organs, acting to accelerate metabolism, lower cholesterol, and other important functions. Thus, low T$_3$ levels in the circulation indicate that the organs contain less T$_3$ than normal, which—based on everything we know about thyroid—leads to reduced T$_3$ action. These findings set the stage for T$_4$-treated patients to exhibit a mild degree of hypothyroidism, despite having normal TSH levels. Could this explain residual hypothyroidism symptoms in some of these patients?

In 2013, I was asked to present some of these studies and pose that question at a conference on hypothyroidism in Washington, DC. I was curious to see the reaction of my colleagues, as it would be the first time I spoke publicly about the body's drive to maintain blood T$_3$ levels. It was also the first time that I remember that someone spoke publicly that patients with hypothyroidism on T$_4$ are not able to maintain circulating-T$_3$ levels—possibly explaining residual symptoms. This was not a concept that many physicians or scientists embraced at the time.

The reaction of the audience was underwhelming. After my presentation, some of my colleagues rightfully argued that even as we accept that T_3 levels are low, a meager 10–15% might not be at all clinically relevant. In other words, such a small drop in T_3 levels might be so small that it is not sufficient to have meaningful consequences.

Well, as we saw, there are two major sets of possible consequences: (1) cognitive, mood, behavior, and quality-of-life symptoms, which are originated in the brain; and (2) metabolic signs and symptoms, which involve multiple organs such as the liver, adipose tissue, muscles, heart, and others. A solid connection between low circulating-T_3 levels and the first set of residual symptoms has not been established. In other words, those patients with the most cognitive symptoms are not the ones with the lowest circulating-T_3 levels.

Even though this question hasn't been looked at consistently, reviewers of my manuscripts constantly remind me that this is a missing link. But they forget good reasons why this might not even be a critical point. For one, circulating-T_3 levels do affect the brain, but they are not the only or even the main factor influencing the brain's T_3 content. The local D2 pathway provides most T_3 in the brain. Thus, issues of cognition, mood, and quality of life, which depend on the T_3 content in the brain, are not exclusively influenced by circulating-T_3 levels. The local D2 pathway and its potential defects play the most important role, confounding the correlation between these symptoms with circulating-T_3 levels.

Studies by Barbara Bocco and her colleagues, while Bocco was a graduate student in my laboratory, illustrate this point. She and other fellows in the lab created a mouse that lacked D2 in the brain. These mice had normal T_3 levels in the circulation—nonetheless, an analysis of their brains revealed a pattern of hypothyroidism. They exhibited anxiety-depression-like behavior.

Thus, despite normal T_3 levels in the blood, a D2 defect in the brain caused behavior modifications compatible with hypothyroidism.[13]

Therefore, any cognitive, mood, behavioral, and quality-of-life symptoms will be greatly influenced by the functionality of the D2 pathway and less so by the T_3 levels in the circulation.

But how about the second set of residual symptoms—the metabolic signs and symptoms? Indeed, as we saw in chapter 9, most T_4-treated patients do have issues with managing body weight, cholesterol levels, and the rate of metabolism. These are likely to be affected primarily by circulating-T_3 levels. The very few clinical trials that looked at this have not found much. But the trials were not designed to measure T_3 as an outcome, meaning they did not have sufficient statistical power to detect relevant differences. I will explain. The methods routinely used to measure T_3 in the blood have technical issues, particularly at the extremes of the normal reference levels. They substantially overestimate low levels of T_3, affecting any correlation with the presence of persistent hypothyroid symptoms. To circumvent this problem, future studies in this area should consider the use of more accurate methods to measure T_3 in the blood. In addition, now that we know that the drop in T_3 levels in patients treated with T_4 is about 10–15%, scientists can calculate the minimum number of patients that must be enrolled in the trial to allow for meaningful conclusions.

In case patients treated with T_3 are to be involved in such studies, the analysis of T_3 levels in blood requires multiple draws within twenty-four hours. In patients taking T_3, circulating levels of T_3 are not steady; they fluctuate substantially due to T_3's rapid absorption and metabolism. Thus, one sample in twenty-four hours does not say much. To have a better assessment of how T_3 levels modify symptoms, we need to calculate "the integrated levels of T_3" over long periods, ideally twenty-four hours.[14]

∗   ∗   ∗

In the late 1970s, as physicians were getting used to treating patients with T_4 and monitoring TSH levels, Chip Ridgway and a dream team of colleagues at Mass General Hospital treated ten patients with hypothyroidism with increasing doses of T_3 for four weeks (10, 25, and 50 micrograms per day for a total of sixteen weeks).[15] Finally, they suspended the administration of T_3, and all patients were switched to 100 to 150 micrograms per day of T_4.

What they found was remarkable: the actions of T_3 in the heart and the skeletal muscles were normalized starting with 20 micrograms per day of T_3, but only 50 micrograms per day of T_3 normalized the body's metabolic rate. Blood cholesterol and TSH levels decreased with T_3 treatment, but neither normalized on any T_3 dose. This confirms that different organs respond differently to circulating T_3 and that small differences in T_3 levels are likely to be clinically relevant.

The next set of results was also surprising. TSH levels normalized upon switching therapy to T_4, but blood T_3 dropped back to the lower limit of the reference range. In addition, the metabolic rate slowed down to subnormal values and blood cholesterol remained elevated. As I mentioned before, T_4 is wonderful for normalizing TSH levels, but not as good when it comes to raising T_3 levels.

Ridgway and his colleagues elegantly demonstrated that a failure to normalize T_3 levels has clear clinical consequences, as these T_4-treated patients persist with a slower metabolism and elevated blood cholesterol. It remains unclear why some organs could be brought back to normal even with subnormal T_3 levels, while other organs and systems remained hypothyroid. It is conceivable that some organs are better equipped to endure thyroid-hormone deficiency. We need to study these mechanisms further.

Though this study was completed more than forty years ago with a small number of patients, the findings support the idea that some patients on T_4 may remain partially hypothyroid—high cholesterol levels and slower metabolism—despite TSH normalization.

* * *

It is disappointing to see how the clinical guidelines prepared by the different professional medical associations ignored the slower metabolism and selectively discussed the issue of low T_3 levels in patients with hypothyroidism treated with T_4. The issue was not mentioned in the 1995 American Thyroid Association guidelines, despite eight studies showing that T_3 was below normal (there were also three studies in which differences could not be detected).[16]

In 2012, the jointly crafted guidelines by the American Thyroid Association and the American Association of Clinical Endocrinology, do talk about it, but selectively rely on a single study that enrolled fifty patients, to state that treatment with T_4 normalizes circulating-T_3 levels.[17] They missed the opportunity to discuss the other nine studies published since 1970 showing that T_3 levels were not normalized in T_4-treated patients.[18] They could have at least said that the issue was not resolved. Most importantly, they also missed a study by Damiano Gullos and his colleagues, published just one year earlier, showing that T_3 levels remained relatively lower during treatment of almost two thousand patients with T_4.[19] Thus, T_4 remained the standard of care of hypothyroidism without any warnings that in many patients T_3 levels were not restored.

* * *

The discovery that the thyroid's primary directive is to sustain normal T_3 levels in the circulation, combined with the inability of T_4 treatment to fully restore thyroid-hormone levels, sparked an awakening. All these studies provide a solid platform for the concept that having lower T_3 levels in the circulation must be clinically relevant. Why physicians (including myself) didn't follow up on the slower metabolism and low T_3 levels of T_4-treated patients much earlier remains a mystery for me. Perhaps the excitement with the discoveries led to an unconscious willingness to overlook anything that could jeopardize the clinical applications of these amazing achievements. After all, the possibility that T_4 alone could be used as therapy for hypothyroidism represented the product of ninety years of discoveries and advancements in the thyroid field.

In the next chapter, I discuss several scenarios to explain why only a minority of the patients treated for hypothyroidism suffer from residual cognitive and quality-of-life symptoms. I give details on how chronic stress and menopausal syndrome can exacerbate and sometimes mimic the residual symptoms of hypothyroidism. But I also detail some of the mechanisms that may be linked to symptoms, such as genetic predisposition, an autoimmune response, even vitamin deficiency. I use my work to explain genetic mechanisms and delve into the details that could play a role in treatment but that are so frequently misunderstood by patients and physicians.

CHAPTER 12

There Is More to Hypothyroidism Than Just Low T₃ Levels

In the winter of 2020, a reporter for a physician website interviewed me on the controversies in the treatment of hypothyroidism. I went to a hotel in downtown Chicago, where a film crew waited for me. It was a chilly morning. The hotel was brand new, a renovation of the beautiful old Cook County Hospital building, where the TV series *ER* was filmed. The building is just next to Rush Hospital, and as I walked down Harrison Street I saw the windows of my old office.

I love to talk, so an interview originally planned for one hour ended up lasting two. As I answered the questions looking toward the camera, I could see the cameraman behind the lights and noticed he was nodding to many of the things I said. I thought to myself, "Does he do this to everybody just to give positive feedback, to assure the speaker? Or is he part of the medical team that formulates the questions?" When I finished with the interview, he approached me and said, "I have hypothyroidism. I have had it since I was seventeen. My doctor put me on T₄ and I have been on the same dose since. I do not feel any of the symptoms you mentioned in your interview. And I never heard that this was a problem to anyone."

Why do some patients on T₄ seem to do so poorly whereas

others are just fine? I know that thyroid-hormone action—T_3 levels—is definitively not normalized in many patients taking T_4. However, why do some patients seem to be particularly sensitive to this? The answer could involve the association with one or more factors.

Indeed, several common conditions unrelated to thyroid disease can disrupt cognition, executive function (the ability to make decisions in a timely fashion), and even humor in ways that resemble hypothyroidism. Chronic stress and the menopausal syndrome (caused by the function of the ovaries shutting down) are examples of such conditions. When combined with the low T_3 levels caused by treatment with T_4, they overload the capacity to adjust or compensate. This occurs because hypothyroidism is so prevalent, it overlaps frequently with other diseases or conditions. It is not uncommon to see a patient on T_4 who is perimenopausal and symptomatic, or a stressed patient who started on T_4 therapy.

In other words, if you have residual symptoms while on therapy with T_4, your doctor should always investigate a possible "two-hit" phenomenon, in which the underlying low T_3 levels are compounded by one or more specific factors that exhaust your ability to compensate.[1] Imagine a condition that would further compromise conversion of T_4 to T_3, or make you more sensitive to problems caused by low T_3 levels. This would intensify the perceived symptoms. Fortunately, this only occurs in a smaller portion of the patients with hypothyroidism.

These additional factors that can interfere with the outcome of T_4 therapy should be in the minds of physicians. For example, when physicians are discussing a potential surgical treatment for a thyroid disease such as a thyroid nodule, the patients should be made aware of the fact that therapy with T_4 might not restore everything to normal, albeit in a small percentage. This fact should enter the decision-making process behind a surgical approach for thyroid disease. It rarely does. Fortunately, most patients know something about it and frequently ask; they might have friends or relatives who are on T_4 therapy.

*   *   *

In T_4-treated patients, most T_3 is produced by the D2 pathway. As we saw, this places D2 in a critical position, which is to define the effectiveness of the therapy with T_4. We know that with the best outcome possible and with a fully functional D2 pathway, T_3 levels will remain at the lower limit of normal or even below normal. Now, here is a question. What would happen if some of the T_4-treated patients had a defect in D2 that further impaired their ability to produce T_3? Would that reduce the T_3 levels in circulation even further? The answer is an emphatic yes. But—for decades—no defects in the D2 pathway had been reported. This has now changed.

*   *   *

A few years ago, Francesco Celi, a clinician-scientist at Virginia Commonwealth University, discovered that many of us carry an inherited polymorphism in the D2 gene.[2] A gene polymorphism is a minor variation from the normal that can occur in a large number of individuals and may affect the function of a protein. The D2 polymorphism identified by Celi is present in up to 45% of the patient sample he studied; a smaller number of individuals have a double dose of the polymorphism. The polymorphism causes an important modification of D2: a change in one of the amino acids—the "building blocks"—in the D2 molecule.

Celi's discovery in 2002 brought excitement to the field. After all, this had been the first time a potential defect had been found with any deiodinase, let alone one involving D2. Through my collaboration with Isabelle Callebaut, we found that all three deiodinases have a very similar structure, but D2 in particular has a unique loop of eighteen amino acids critical for its tagging and destruction. Remarkably, position 92, where Celi located the polymorphism, is the first amino acid in that loop, placing it at a critical location to affect the D2 pathway.[3]

Of course, we were not the only group looking at this. Worldwide, scientists were asking the same questions, and unfortunately, none (including us) could find a functional difference between the normal D2 and the polymorphic D2. This was disappointing, but not final.

In just a few years, a new study changed everything.[4] Colin Dayan and his group looked at whether being a carrier of the D2 polymorphism affects the way a patient responds to treatment with T_4. He studied 550 patients with hypothyroidism and assessed their quality-of-life and other thyroid-related symptoms using questionnaires. Dayan discovered that carriers of the D2 polymorphism exhibited worse psychological well-being and were more likely to have signs of depression. They also found that carriers of the D2 polymorphism responded positively to combination therapy containing $T_4 + T_3$.

These findings were so exciting that I almost immediately embarked on a long-term project to create a new mouse model that carried the polymorphic human D2 gene. This mouse would allow me to go much deeper into the effects of the polymorphic D2 on behavior, mood, cognition, and metabolism.

* * *

A couple of years later, the mice were ready. We were enthusiastic, but couldn't find anything wrong with them. Nothing. The mice grew and gained weight as expected, and reproduced normally. Their thyroid glands seemed fine, of normal size, and the circulating levels of TSH, T_4, and T_3 were within normal range.

Next, we tested their metabolism. But again, they had a normal metabolic rate, even when exposed to cold, which is a way we use in the laboratory to accelerate the metabolic rate. They responded just like the control mice. One more test was to see how well these mice could handle a high-fat diet, which normally causes obesity in mice. They did well. Again, no differences were observed when the results of the polymorphic D2 mice were compared to mice having the normal D2 gene.

All these experiments took years to complete, along with monumental effort and many resources. Students in particular get frustrated and lose interest when nothing exciting is found right away. As it turns out, we of course were looking in the wrong place. So, when we were just about to give up, I spoke to Miriam Ribeiro, the scientist at MacKenzie Presbyterian University, and she suggested we study the mice's behavior, mood, and cognition—after all, the chief complaints of the patients seemed to be around these areas. (This seems so obvious now!)

Under her guidance, we set the mice in special cages, where they had free access to food and water and were monitored 24/7, with the help of light beams and a computer. The results were dramatic.[5] The control mice moved about 850 feet in forty-eight hours, whereas the mice carrying the polymorphic D2 gene moved only about 600 feet during the same period. In addition, they slept at least four times more than the control mice! We figured that perhaps they were bored. We then installed a spinning wheel inside each cage so that the mice could spin and play. The polymorphic D2 mice used the wheel half as much as the control mice! We repeated this several times and always saw the same results.

Additional studies revealed that the polymorphic D2 mice

stayed quiet when left alone but, when prompted, responded to stimuli even more than the control mice. For example, when placed in a new environment, they moved and sniffed around; when placed in a maze, they explored for longer times, taking chances. But after a few minutes, they lost interest and went back to sleep. We reasoned that these animals could be depressed. Yes, perhaps depression made them not want to play and quickly lose interest in things. They were tested, but no sign of depression could be identified.

Then we tested their memory, and voilà! We found a major problem. We showed them objects of different forms for only five minutes. Three and twenty-four hours later, they were retested to see if they recalled what they saw. The polymorphic D2 mice had no short-term memory at all.

To explain these results, we hypothesized that although the bodies of the polymorphic D2 mice seemed fine, their brains had localized hypothyroidism. In theory, this was possible because, as shown many years before by Enrique Silva and Reed Larsen, most T_3 in the brain is produced locally by the D2 pathway. The brain does have access to T_3 from the circulation, but D2 in the brain is so active that it ends up inundating the brain with locally produced T_3. Well, if D2 is so important for the brain, then it makes sense that the polymorphic D2 mice would have the most symptoms connected with behavior and cognition.

Support for this theory came from Domenico Salvatore, a physician-scientist at the University of Naples. Salvatore and I became friends in 1998 when he was a fellow in Reed Larsen's laboratory. After his fellowship in Boston, Salvatore went back to Naples, where he leads a group of thyroid scientists. There, he used an improved system to measure the ability of D2 to generate T_3 through its downstream effects. He obtained strong evidence that polymorphic D2 is slower than normal at producing T_3.[6] This was a very important finding that could explain Colin Dayan's results as well as the behavior of the polymorphic D2 mice we had created in the lab.

I reviewed Salvatore's data with great enthusiasm, and—using a similar, more direct method—we found out that the polymorphic D2 produces about 20% less T_3 than the normal D2 enzyme.[7] Indeed, these findings explained the bizarre behavior of our polymorphic D2 mice. The atypical enzyme produces less T_3. Because the brain relies on T_3 that is produced locally by D2, above all other organs, the brain suffers more.

Our next move was to zero in on the brains of the polymorphic D2 mice. We took them apart and studied the expression of all known genes, about thirty thousand. Soon after, we identified a few abnormalities. The analysis revealed that thyroid-hormone action was slightly diminished in three areas: the prefrontal cortex (an area involved in decision-making processes), the striatum (an area involved in motivation and initiation of activities), and the hippocampus (an area involved with memory processes). Most important, these animals had a normal TSH level and yet had brain hypothyroidism, with cognitive impairment and behavior that resembled that of T_4-treated patients with residual symptoms.

To close the loop and provide even stronger support for our findings, we "treated" the polymorphic D2 mice with T_3 for just ten days—to force T_3 into their brains and eliminate brain hypothyroidism. To our amazement, they recovered from all behavior and cognitive abnormalities.

Next, we made the polymorphic D2 mice hypothyroid, simply by giving them water containing an antithyroid medication. After they became hypothyroid, we treated them with a daily oral dose of T_4 that normalized their TSH levels. We wanted to reproduce what is done to patients with hypothyroidism. While the control mice responded well to therapy with T_4, with normal behavior and cognitive function, the polymorphic D2 mice only had a partial response, exhibiting clues of residual brain hypothyroidism. Combination therapy with T_4 and T_3 fixed the problem.

*   *   *

The results obtained in the D2 polymorphic mice were thrilling. They provided a fascinating insight into what could be happening in the brain of some T_4-treated patients. But how could we test the brains of patients carrying the D2 polymorphism?

When I was working in Miami, I established a collaboration with Deborah Mash, a scientist and the director of the Brain Endowment Bank at the University of Miami. Through Mash, I gained access to brains from relatively young individuals who died as a result of trauma, such as car accidents or gunshot wounds. This allowed us to study the brains of relatively healthy people with no known neurological or thyroid diseases. Mash prepared brain samples from about a hundred individuals, and Elizabeth McAninch in my group identified the ones with D2 polymorphism.

Similar to what we did to the mice, McAninch looked at gene expression in the brains of these individuals and discovered that carriers of the D2 polymorphism exhibited signs of cellular distress.[8] These findings were reminiscent of what is seen in the brains of patients with neurodegenerative disorders such as Alzheimer's or Parkinson's disease.

Of course, we looked for confirmation of these findings and decided to use a human cell line in culture. We modified these cells to express either the normal D2 or the polymorphic D2. Then we compared both batches of cells. Again, we found clear signs of cellular stress in the cells expressing the polymorphic D2 gene, like what we saw in the human and mouse brains. What could be causing these abnormalities?

I spoke to Balázs Gereben in Budapest and asked him to look

at these cells using an electron microscope, which is a very powerful tool to look at details of the internal structures of a cell. He worked with his colleague Csaba Fekete, also a scientist in Budapest, and found the normal D2 located where it was supposed to be (around the cell nucleus). However, they saw that the polymorphic D2 was elsewhere—in the Golgi apparatus, a cellular structure involved in the processing and transporting of cell proteins. D2 was not supposed to be there. Not a single time did they see normal D2 in the Golgi.[9]

Investigating further, we discovered that the amino acid substitution causes D2 to misfold. And the misfolded D2 accumulated in the cells, causing stress. In general, when misfolded proteins accumulate, cells try to get rid of them by using the proteasome system (the vacuum cleaner that destroys proteins inside cells; see chapter 10). But in the case of D2, the change in amino acid made it less susceptible to this route, and the cells reacted by pushing it away to the Golgi apparatus, which then affected its normal function.

We went back to the brains of the individuals carrying the D2 polymorphism and found alterations in dozens of Golgi-related genes.[10] This is indeed fascinating, as we know that the brains of patients with Alzheimer's disease also exhibit an accumulation of misfolded protein in the Golgi apparatus.

*   *   *

Could it be possible that the polymorphic D2 causes brain degeneration, similar to what Alzheimer's patients have? To answer that question, I spoke to Denis Evans, a physician-scientist in Chicago, at the time leading a program known as the Rush Institute for Healthy Aging. This program followed thousands of individuals who underwent a complete annual neurological assessment performed by a neurologist. Evans gave us access to data in community-based cohorts from Chicago and northeastern Illinois, as well as clergymen from across the United States.

Elizabeth McAninch examined this data and asked whether having the D2 polymorphism affects the likelihood of developing Alzheimer's disease or other forms of dementia. We know that African Americans are more likely to develop these conditions, so we analyzed about 3,000 African Americans and 9,300 European Americans separately.

McAninch found no association between the D2 polymorphism and Alzheimer's disease in European Americans.[11] In contrast, she found that African American carriers of the D2 polymorphism had 1.3 times greater odds of developing Alzheimer's. A secondary analysis of a representative sample of the United States population revealed that African American carriers of the D2 polymorphism had increased odds of dementia and 1.35 times greater odds of developing cognitive impairment.

We don't know why the association was observed only in African Americans. Because African Americans have a greater likelihood of developing Alzheimer's disease, it is conceivable that the effects of D2 polymorphism are easier to detect in those who are already predisposed to the disease.

There is still a lot to learn in this area. For example, why are healthy carriers of the D2 polymorphism (that is, those with a normal thyroid gland) reportedly asymptomatic when surveyed through the quality-of-life or thyroid-specific questionnaires? Why have abnormalities been reported only in connection with diagnosis and treatment for hypothyroidism?

As discussed earlier, carriers of the D2 polymorphism have the potential to adapt to and minimize cognitive defects through lifelong learning and training. This is called intellectual enrichment. However, once adult carriers of the D2 polymorphism become hypothyroid and are treated with T_4, these adaptive mechanisms could be exhausted, bringing out some of the symptoms we observed in the polymorphic D2 mice. The approximately 10% lower T_3 levels observed in conventionally T_4-treated patients could be the key element that tips the balance toward cognitive dysfunction.

Multiple centers around the world reported studies of the association or lack thereof between the D2 polymorphism and several diseases and conditions. So far, the results have been marked by inconsistency.[12] Apart from involving only a small number of patients—which limits the power to detect statistical differences—association studies of gene polymorphisms in humans are in general less powerful because of differences in the genetic background among individuals. Thus, it is understandable that the effects of D2 polymorphism depend on the population that is being studied and that data obtained across the world may be conflicting.

*   *   *

As I have said many times throughout this book, it is clear that the success of the treatment with T_4 depends on the deiodinases, which activate T_4-to-T_3 conversion. The available data indicates that the D2 is the critical enzyme that produces most T_3 in T_4-treated patients. In contrast, the D1 pathway does not seem to be as critical. Like the D2 pathway, D1 is a deiodinase that can convert T_4-to-T_3. However, D1 is a "lazy" enzyme, not as efficient as D2. As a result, T_4 is pulled toward D2 and the amount of T_4 that ends up going through the D1 pathway is a lot less, only about 20%.

Nonetheless, a defect in the D1 pathway could still play a role in T_4-treated patients, compromising the activation of T_4 to T_3, especially if this defect is combined with a D2 polymorphism in the same patient.

Robin Peeters and I worked together in Boston when he was a

fellow in Reed Larsen's laboratory. At that time we studied how, during iodine deficiency, the deiodinases in the brain adapt to preserve T_3 action. Peeters went back to the Erasmus University in Rotterdam, the Netherlands, where he leads a team of thyroid scientists and, among other things, studies large sets of patients looking for genetic variability that could explain greater susceptibility to thyroid disease.

Peeters and his group identified a series of D1 gene polymorphisms that could be clinically relevant in patients treated with T_4.[13] There is evidence that at least one of these polymorphisms may compromise D1's ability to convert T_4 to T_3. In addition, as discussed earlier, Alexandra Dumitrescu and Samuel Refetoff at the University of Chicago identified a few families that carried mutations in D1.[14] The mutations resulted in a defective enzyme with much slower activity—about 50% less—than the control enzyme.

These genetic abnormalities in the deiodinase pathways go unnoticed in individuals with a normal thyroid gland because of adjustments in thyroidal T_3 secretion that defends T_3 levels. However, in patients with hypothyroidism treated with T_4, carrying D1 and/or D2 abnormalities is very likely to result in reduced circulating levels of T_3. There is much to be learned about the genetic makeup of patients with hypothyroidism who remain symptomatic on T_4.

* * *

An autoimmune disease is a condition in which your immune system mistakenly attacks your body. The immune system normally produces antibodies to defend against invading organisms, such as bacteria and viruses that cause diseases. Under normal circumstances, the immune system easily distinguishes your own cells from foreign cells, sending cells and antibodies to kill them.

If you have an autoimmune condition, it is because your immune system has lost the ability to distinguish some of your cells from foreign ones. Consequently, it unleashes an immune attack that interferes with or destroys your healthy cells.

If the immune response targets the pancreas, you may lose the ability to produce insulin and may develop type 1 diabetes. In other cases, like systemic lupus erythematosus, autoantibodies attack multiple organs in the body at the same time. There is a great deal of variability among patients regarding how this immune response actually plays out. For example, certain ethnic groups are more frequently affected by specific autoimmune diseases, such as lupus in African Americans and Hispanic individuals. Furthermore, certain autoimmune diseases run in families. This does not mean that every family member will have the same disease. It means that family members will inherit a greater susceptibility and thus are more likely to develop an autoimmune condition.

Having an autoimmune disease, such as Hashimoto's disease, increases the risk of developing a second or third autoimmune condition. In other words, patients are commonly affected by two or more autoimmune conditions, which can occur up to 25% of the time. Some combinations of autoimmune conditions are more frequent than others. For example, multiple sclerosis is associated with autoimmune thyroid disease and psoriasis. Type 1 diabetes is associated with several autoimmune conditions and—above all—hypothyroidism.

Many of the autoimmune conditions associated with Hashimoto's disease can cause cognitive symptoms, sometimes even without the patient's knowledge. A condition known as Hashimoto's encephalopathy is a good example of how this may happen.[15] This is a rare disease characterized by impaired brain function (encephalopathy). The exact cause is unknown, but it is believed to result from abnormal functioning of the immune system. It is a powerful example of how autoantibodies linked to thyroid autoimmunity might affect cognition, independently of thyroid-hormone levels.

Patients with Hashimoto's disease have higher levels of auto-antibodies directed against specific parts of the brain, and this might have functional consequences.[16] For example, using sophisticated imaging techniques, physicians have identified a reduction in the brain's blood perfusion in a group of patients with Hashimoto's disease who had normal TSH levels and a normal neurological examination.[17] This is important because blood flow brings oxygen and nutrients to the brain, which ensures normal brain function. In another study, physicians used MRI spectroscopy to study T_4-treated patients with Hashimoto's disease and found abnormal levels of certain cerebral metabolites, which can lead to a reduction of brain activity, despite normal TSH levels.[18]

Altogether, these findings raise the possibility that some patients with Hashimoto's disease might have reduced blood flow to the brain. Unfortunately, considering these elements in assessing the effectiveness of therapy with T_4 in clinical practice is not always feasible, as it requires time, resources, and the utilization of advanced diagnostic tools.

Other low-grade autoimmune conditions that do not target the brain per se can also lead to cognitive dysfunction and nonspecific symptoms that resemble those of hypothyroidism. For example, even prior to the development of anemia, a deficiency in vitamin B12 can cause numbness or tingling in the extremities; balance problems; cognitive impairment such as difficulty thinking and reasoning, or memory loss; weakness; or fatigue.[19] In fact, B12 deficiency is prevalent among patients with Hashimoto's disease because of the association with two other conditions—atrophic gastritis and pernicious anemia—both leading to impaired B12 absorption. Atrophic gastritis is present in 35–40% of patients with Hashimoto's disease and pernicious anemia in 16%.[20]

Thus, there is much to consider when assessing patients with hypothyroidism who remain symptomatic despite treatment with T$_4$. While there is room for improvement in the way we plan treatment for hypothyroidism, it is undeniable that concomitant diseases can contribute to residual symptoms and must be explored. When found, they must be appropriately addressed.

* * *

Treatment of hypothyroidism is not as simple as we physicians or patients have been told. Many more things need to be considered in addition to circulating levels of TSH. The next part of the book presents the latest clinical science on combination treatment and what can be done today to optimize the treatment of hypothyroidism. It includes a discussion of the clinical trials and whether combination therapy works, if it is safe, and how it is done; and finally, of what is in the pipeline in terms of new treatments for hypothyroidism.

PART FIVE

The Treatments

CHAPTER 13

Understanding Combination Therapy

In the preceding chapters, I have built a case that the switch to treating patients with synthetic T_4 along with adjustments of the dose based on TSH levels led to insufficient production of T_3, the hormone that resolves symptoms in hypothyroid patients. In other words, the levels of T_3 are not fully replenished by treatment with T_4. Low T_3 levels can contribute to the cognitive, mood, and metabolic residual symptoms experienced by some of the T_4-treated patients. It is conceivable that the genetic makeup of each patient and the presence of other chronic diseases or conditions, including whether the patient is menopausal, could play additional roles as well. For now, adjusting low T_3 levels seem to be the low-hanging fruit.

Scientists found in the 1970s that T_3 production does not return to normal in many T_4-treated patients. As we discussed, patient complaints made some physicians skeptical of switching to T_4. Instead, they continued treating patients with thyroid extract. In addition, these physicians also treated patients with combination therapy—two tablets—containing T_4 + T_3. Anecdotally, many patients felt better with thyroid extract or combination therapy. But is this sufficient to treat all patients with hypothyroidism with combination therapy?

*　*　*

A fundamental aspect of modern medicine is to use evidence-based principles to guide the diagnosis and treatment of diseases. When a physician prescribes a therapy to a patient, they assure the patient that the therapy has been tested without bias and that the results were positive. In general, there are always risks; but the hallmark of any good therapy is that the benefits outweigh the risks by a significant margin.

The clinical trial is central to evidence-based medicine. A good trial is a coordinated and systematic study of a group of patients for a predetermined number of weeks, months, or years, during which scientists monitor the effects of an intervention. Key features of a clinical trial include:

- A sufficient number of patients to allow meaningful conclusions based on rigorous statistical analysis. This is determined through "power analysis," which depends on the clinical parameters that will be monitored during a trial, and the expected changes. For example, at the end of the trial, scientists will determine with certainty that a specific intervention lowered blood pressure by 10%. Other examples of typical parameters assessed during a clinical trial are body weight, questionnaires, or imaging studies (any of which could substantiate the outcome(s) of the trial).
- The blind randomization of patients between the intervention and control groups. This means patients are randomized to either group, and no one in the study—including patients, doctors, nurses, and others—knows which group each participant is assigned to.

So, when I prescribe T_4, I assure my patients that, based on solid historical data and some clinical studies, most patients with hypothyroidism (anywhere between 80–90%) respond well to the medication, signs and symptoms of overt hypothyroidism should be eliminated, and the risks of taking the medication are negligent. I also tell them that about 10–20% of the patients continue with symptoms in areas such as cognition, mood, and quality of life. Lastly, I tell them that we know of residual metabolic abnormalities that affect all T_4-treated patients, such as the tendency to gain weight, lower metabolic rates, and elevated cholesterol levels.

The conversation around combination therapy is not as simple. Yes, combination therapy is also based on solid historical data—largely from the use of thyroid extract—but very few clinical studies. It does eliminate signs and symptoms of overt hypothyroidism, and the risks are probably negligent. However, because the use of thyroid extract was all but abandoned after the 1980s, these conclusions are based more on clinical experience and expert opinion than on objective clinical trials.

Nonetheless, there were clinical trials comparing monotherapy (use of T_4 only) with combination therapy (use of $T_4 + T_3$). But, unfortunately, these trials enrolled patients with hypothyroidism indistinctively, not just those who remain symptomatic after treatment with T_4. Studying eighteen clinical trials that involved almost a thousand patients with hypothyroidism while on T_4 or $T_4 + T_3$ for up to one year, a multinational group of scientists analyzed the effectiveness of each therapy and patient preferences.[1]

The trials' designers randomly assigned patients to either monotherapy or combination therapy. In other trials, after several weeks on T_4 and without anyone knowing, the trial designers switched patients to $T_4 + T_3$ (or vice versa), where they remained for the same amount of time. In all trials, the designers adjusted the doses of combination therapy based on TSH levels, which remained within normal range. In general, patients received reduced doses of T_4 to allow for the addition of T_3. Using the TSH levels to adjust the doses in each treatment group ensured that both therapies were equivalent and the combination therapy did not result in an excessive or insufficient dose of thyroid hormones.

As expected, patients on combination therapy exhibited an improved profile of thyroid-hormone levels; T_4 levels were no longer elevated, and T_3 levels were restored—well within normal range—while maintaining normal TSH levels. To tell which therapy was better, physicians used questionnaires designed to evaluate dozens of parameters about mood, cognition, energy level, and quality of life.

After all the data was computed, most clinical trials did not show superiority of combination therapy or monotherapy on clinical status, quality of life, psychological distress, depressive symptoms, and fatigue; all measured with standardized questionnaires and compared with patients taking T_4 only.

Indeed, when enrolling *all patients with hypothyroidism*, therapies with T_4 or $T_4 + T_3$ have been repeatedly shown to be equivalent in terms of efficacy and frequency of adverse events. Thus, when also considering cost and convenience, professional guidelines have argued that, as a group, patients with hypothyroidism are better served by treatment with T_4 only.

* * *

It is important to note that studying the quality of life and mood requires asking questions that might have nonobjective answers—for example, "What is your level of sadness?" as opposed to "Are your fasting blood glucose levels at 95 mg/dl?" The nature of the questions makes the answers susceptible to nonspecific influences, which makes it hard to perform a robust comparative analysis between studies and between therapies. Thus, it can be difficult to pinpoint if improvement or decline in any of these aspects is due to a superior thyroid-hormone treatment, or if changes took place because of what happened with an associated condition, or some of the other known or unknown confounders.

All of this can be addressed in the design of the clinical trial, but addressing it properly requires large numbers of patients, to increase the statistical power for finding differences between the two treatments. This increases the cost of the trial. Further, it is very difficult to obtain funds for trials that aim at improving the treatment of hypothyroidism because the dogma is that this issue was resolved fifty years ago. I hear this frequently, and as recently as a few months ago before writing this chapter, in a panel of experts ranking research proposals, someone asked, "Why are we even considering this proposal if there is a cheap and effective treatment for hypothyroidism?"

Now, here is a parameter that is slightly more objective and easier to assess: What do the trials say about preference? The clinical trials indicate a patient preference for combination therapy, even when the trials are blinded, randomized, and placebo controlled. This means patients prefer combination therapy even as the questionnaires are not able to capture the reason(s). In an analysis, the multinational group of scientists identified higher proportions of preference choice for combined therapy (~45%) when compared to monotherapy (~25%) or having no preference (30%).

For reasons I do not quite understand, patient preference has only briefly been mentioned and has not been considered when issuing guidelines on the treatment of hypothyroidism. If the trials conducted so far show that T_4 or $T_4 + T_3$ are equivalent, then why not favor combination therapy based on preference? I asked my colleagues that exact question and remain unconvinced by their answer. They seem to think that if the preference is real, then a reason for it should have been captured in the questionnaires.

I am puzzled by this. This is like telling someone you prefer lemonade instead of orange juice. Then you are given multiple questionnaires to understand why you prefer lemonade, but the questionnaires do not quite capture an explanation. That doesn't mean you actually prefer orange juice; it means you were asked the wrong questions.

Specialists in the design of clinical trials are aware of the gap that exists between patient preference and patient-reported outcomes (recorded in questionnaires). The latter may lack the ability to capture information that patients rank as most important in their daily life. In other words, we are simply not asking the right questions. As a result, patients may not be achieving outcomes that are meaningful to them; patient and physician goals may be misaligned—for example, quality of life versus TSH levels. In addition, what I hear from my colleagues is that many do not consider patient preference when engaging in shared decision-making conversations.

Many approaches have been studied to bridge this gap, including the "treat-to-target" (or T2T) approach, largely focused on the development of tools that track and score a patient's experience with their perception of symptoms.

The key take-home message is that if the consensus is that T_4 and $T_4 + T_3$ therapies are equivalent, then patient preference must be brought to the forefront of patient care. Patient preference must be considered as a valid outcome in future clinical trials, given its strength and simplicity to obtain. Not doing so perpetuates the idea that physicians do not listen to or do disregard patients' opinions. It seems that a more holistic approach focused on clinical outcomes, patient-reported outcomes, and patient preferences should be adopted when crafting clinical guidelines to treat chronic diseases, including hypothyroidism.

*　*　*

So, as a group, therapy with T_4 is equivalent to therapy with T_4 and T_3 when cognition, mood, and quality of life are considered. But patients demonstrably tend to prefer combination therapy over T_4. In addition, on a case-by-case basis, some patients unequivocally benefit from combination therapy. Keeping in mind that most patients do just fine on T_4 alone, and that combination therapy is not a panacea that works for every symptomatic patient, one can't help but wonder why physicians are not more liberal in prescribing combination therapy based on individual preference.

An incomplete long-term safety record has been mentioned as an issue associated with the use of T_3, which gives physicians pause. After taking a tablet of T_3 or thyroid extract, T_3 is rapidly absorbed into the circulation, and, after two to three hours, a spike of T_3 can be detected. T_3 levels can increase as much as 50%, or even more depending on the dose of T_3 in the tablet. About twenty hours after this spike, T_3 returns to baseline levels. It is a roller coaster.

At the T_3 peak level, patients might feel better but could also complain of palpitations in the chest and neck, chest tightness, sweating, fine tremor, or feeling jittery. Most patients do not present these adverse reactions, which depend on the patient and the dose of T_3. High levels of T_3 could potentially increase the likelihood of atrial fibrillation and osteoporosis—two very serious conditions.

Thus, a factor that should be weighed when considering combination therapy is a concern with those spikes of T_3 in the circulation. These risks are real, especially in older individuals. That said, as with any medication, T_4, T_3, and thyroid extract have their recommended doses and indications. If used above the recommended dose or when it is not indicated, it becomes dangerous, just like with any other drug.

In all fairness, aside from a theoretical risk, is there a solid basis for safety concerns with T_3 or thyroid extract? Since this concern is stated in every guideline and highlighted by many physicians, I have always been under the impression that it was based on facts. Around 2017, I started looking for studies in which these facts would have been documented but could not find a single one. Then I asked Thayer Idrees, a clinical fellow in my group, to perform a systematic search of all studies in which T_3 or thyroid extract had been administered to humans. What he found (or could not find) surprised me.

All clinical trials indicate that the combination of T_4 with T_3 to treat hypothyroidism is safe and effective. In these trials, the combination therapy was introduced by replacing a fraction of the dose of T_4 with T_3, while maintaining TSH levels *within normal range*. The spikes of circulating T_3 observed after the T_3 tablets only minimally affected TSH, heart rate, and blood pressure; the frequency of adverse reactions was similar to patients taking T_4 alone. Markers of bone metabolism were elevated in patients on combination therapy, but well within the normal reference range. There were very few adverse reactions reported, and their frequency was similar in both forms of treatment.

In my mind, an amazing study published a few years ago puts the issue of T_3 safety to rest. During 1997 and 2014 in the Scottish region of Tayside, physicians looked at thousands of individuals for an average of about nine years. They identified about thirty-four thousand patients taking T_4 only, and compared them with about four hundred patients taking T_4 + T_3 or T_3 alone. They observed no differences in mortality or morbidity risk due to cardiovascular disease, atrial fibrillation, or fractures when the three groups were compared. A subsequent study included all adult individuals living in Sweden who used thyroid hormone between July 2005 and December 2017 (a little over a half-million people). They concluded that the use of T_3 by approximately eleven thousand individuals during a median follow-up time of about eight years did not increase all-cause mortality compared with T_4 use.[2]

Safety data on T_3-containing therapy obtained from all published clinical trials does not give reasons for concerns. Nonetheless, one should keep in mind that most clinical trials to date recruited only uncomplicated patients with hypothyroidism— namely, those who were not pregnant or breastfeeding, patients without cardiovascular preconditions, or patients concomitantly receiving other drugs that could amplify many of the T_3-dependent biological effects. Nothing can be said about safety in these more complicated cases.

*   *   *

As we have seen throughout this book, the use of animal-thyroid extracts developed in the 1890s is also a form of combination therapy that includes T_4 and T_3. Thyroid extract is a non-FDA-approved form of combination therapy in which the relative amounts of T_4 and T_3 are fixed at a relatively higher level of T_3, 4:1. That means patients on thyroid extract take slightly more T_3 than they would otherwise take using a combination of T_4 with T_3 formulated by their doctors. Again, given the availability of synthetic $T_4 + T_3$ as well as the paucity of information about the shelf life of the different brands of thyroid extracts, I normally prefer not to start patients on thyroid extract. However, I recognize that many patients have a preference for and do well on thyroid extract. For those patients, I would normally refill their prescriptions after I was satisfied that the dose was right (checking the TSH levels) and the patients were not experiencing signs or symptoms of excessive treatment.

There are a few trials that have studied thyroid extract in the treatment of hypothyroidism with an observational period of about two years.[3] Some manufacturers are currently working with the FDA on large clinical trials to obtain full FDA approval. Typically, thyroid extract resolves symptoms of hypothyroidism with no adverse reactions, as long as TSH levels are used to adjust the dose. But the long-term assessment of the treatment's effects on bone metabolism hasn't been done.

The mean daily dose needed to bring TSH levels back to the reference range contains about 11 micrograms of T_3; some patients may require higher doses of thyroid extract, which can bring the daily T_3 dose to about 24 micrograms. While these doses are more likely to elevate T_3 levels temporarily above the normal reference range, patients have not exhibited adverse reactions in clinical trials in which TSH levels were maintained within normal range.

Professional societies do not endorse the use of thyroid extract, given the limited long-term safety data, the extract's relatively higher content of T_3, and its historical inconsistency of potency. Nonetheless, physicians are placing an increasing number of patients on thyroid extract. Using Marketscan—a tool to investigate insurance claims on all prescriptions in the United States—Matt Ettleson, a clinical fellow in my group, estimated that between the late 2010s and early 2020s there were about 1.5 million patients on thyroid extract, whereas the number on combination therapy with T_4 and T_3 was about four hundred thousand. This is quite remarkable.

In the summer of 2018, an MIT undergrad, Sabrina Ibarra, worked in my laboratory. I asked her and Sarah Peterson, the clinical nutritionist at Rush Hospital with whom I collaborated in the past, to identify parameters in the NHANES database that could explain why thyroid extract remains so popular. (As I mentioned earlier, NHANES collects social and health data from individuals across the country and stores it in a publicly available database.)

In just a few days, Ibarra and Peterson had made a startling discovery: Patients on thyroid extract maintain a much "healthier" lifestyle when compared to patients on T_4. They exercise more. Their diet contains more fiber, polyunsaturated fatty acids, plain water, nuts/seeds, vegetables, and legumes, and less milk and yogurt. Their diets also contain more carotenes and folate, and they take more vitamins and minerals as dietary supplements. Ibarra and Peterson also noticed that those patients have a smaller waist circumference, higher vitamin D levels, and lower hemoglobin A1c levels (a metabolic index indicating diabetes) and use fewer of any other prescription medications.

The marketing of thyroid extract weighs heavily on the fact that it is the "natural" treatment for hypothyroidism. Some commercial brands include the word *natural* in their brand names. Many of my patients explicitly refused to take anything synthetic (for example, T_4 or T_3), as they prefer something natural like thyroid extract. Popular social media discussion groups for patients with hypothyroidism also talk about the perceived benefit of natural versus synthetic thyroid hormones all the time. Thus, the fact that thyroid extract is an animal product ends up being an inherent appeal to those patients who have a compatible lifestyle.

It is conceivable that thyroid extract is the preferred treatment of patients who are focused on eating nutritious food. The data also suggest that these individuals exhibit a higher level of "nature connectedness"—in other words, the extent to which individuals include nature as part of their identity. Nature connectedness is similar to a personality trait: it is stable over time and across various situations. It can help us cope with stress and fatigue, which as we saw is a key residual symptom of T_4-treated patients. Studies in environmental psychology suggest that a connection with nature may serve an adaptive function, psychological restoration.[4]

It is thus possible that some patients are better equipped to cope with residual symptoms due to their higher level of nature connectedness. And for them, preferring thyroid extract is linked to this trait. If this is confirmed, it would indicate that the combination of T_4 with T_3 in thyroid extract might not be the only element that makes some patients prefer thyroid extract.

*   *   *

So, what is the way out of this conundrum about current treatments of hypothyroidism? Many patients guarantee they prefer and feel better on combination therapy, either synthetic $T_4 + T_3$ or thyroid extract. And yet, almost twenty clinical trials were not able to capture these differences while considering the whole group of patients with hypothyroidism. How is this possible? As we will see in the next chapter, in many cases we were asking the wrong questions to the wrong group of patients. Things became very clear once we figured this out and performed the first double-blind randomized clinical trial to compare the three leading forms of treatment for hypothyroidism: T_4 versus $T_4 + T_3$ versus thyroid extract.

CHAPTER 14

Embracing Options

The preceding chapters gave you an idea of what was going through my mind when, in the summer of 2011, I started working with Jacquie Jonklaas, the clinician-scientist at Georgetown University, on a task force to craft the 2014 American Thyroid Association guidelines. The group felt that substantial progress had been made in the basic sciences arena, which was not on the radar of clinicians treating patients with hypothyroidism. To capture this, several leading experts reviewed thousands of publications, and, for the first time in our area, recommendations were based on clinical as well as scientific rationales.[1]

This was a deliberate attempt to refocus the discussion on science, bridging the gap that naturally exists between the scientists and the doctors who focus mostly on patient care. We hoped scientists reading the document would be made aware of the clinical problems that needed to be tackled, and the clinicians would learn more about the advances in our understanding of the thyroid-hormone metabolism and action.

The task force had to consider mounting scientific evidence of residual symptoms of hypothyroidism despite normal TSH levels, that T_3 levels remained low in T_4-treated patients, and that the prolonged use of T_3 seemed safe from the study data. So, the group was willing to substantially modify the association's recommendations issued just two years earlier. Much like the European guidelines, the resulting 2014 American Thyroid Association document recognized:

- Some T_4-treated patients remain symptomatic despite appropriate treatment.
- Circulating levels of T_3 are relatively low and might not even be normalized in all T_4-treated patients. This was a critical point given that it officially recognizes that treatment with T_4 does not restore the levels of the active thyroid hormone—that is, T_3, the one that is capable of resolving symptoms of hypothyroidism.
- More studies were needed to define the clinical significance of lower T_3 levels in T_4-treated patients.
- Combination therapy with T_4 + T_3 is not a panacea and should not be used as a routine approach to patients with hypothyroidism. It should be attempted on a trial basis for those 10–20% of patients with hypothyroidism who undoubtedly do not benefit fully from T_4. Hence, the door was opened for physicians to start combination therapy on most patients with hypothyroidism who felt dissatisfied with T_4.
- The pharmaceutical companies could mobilize and develop new ways to administer T_3 without causing much fluctuation in its circulating levels.

After the guidelines were published, I went online and looked for patients' reactions in blogs and discussion groups. There were criticisms, and I can understand. For many, this was too little, too late. If you have hypothyroidism and became symptomatic after the switch to T_4 during the 1970s, you had to come to terms with the fact that it took about fifty years for the American Thyroid Association to recognize and address your problem—and despite all the evidence that was available since 1970. A major reckoning is in order, and, in my view, apologies as well.

* * *

Following the 2014 American Thyroid Association guidelines, physicians in the United States started to talk openly about combination therapy for hypothyroidism. The next milestone that paved the pathway toward seriously considering alternatives to treatment with T$_4$ was the online survey, which I mentioned earlier.[2] The survey attached real numbers to the vague idea that patients with hypothyroidism were unhappy. Similar to the letters written by patients to Naomi Roberts in the United Kingdom, thousands of patients consistently complained bitterly about very similar issues, about their treatments and being ignored by physicians. It is not a patient conspiracy. It is much more likely that they feel as bad as they said they do.

While this did not come as a surprise to many of us who see patients with hypothyroidism, these real numbers made a big impact. And for many people involved in the world of hypothyroidism, seeing so much dissatisfaction with physicians was eye-opening. Yes, there was immediate pushback from colleagues related to the survey itself. I heard it all. One comment indicative of refusal to acknowledge fault was: "Oh yes, we knew about this—there is nothing new in this survey. These represent the emotionally unstable patients with hypothyroidism."

Nonetheless, in the end, the most important information collected by this survey was the objective knowledge that thousands, perhaps millions, of patients with hypothyroidism are dissatisfied with their treatment and their doctors. I am confident that these results helped move the physicians' perspective. I have witnessed many physicians now openly discussing and considering the clinical entity of a dissatisfied patient with hypothyroidism kept on T$_4$.

Like them, I felt that too. While a few years ago I was uncomfortable bringing up the issue of residual symptoms from patients on T_4 at a professional meeting or even with my colleagues, after the survey results were published it became clear that this topic is here to stay. I also believe that the survey results prompted the American Thyroid Association and other professional societies to review their stance. They realized what a missed opportunity this was and that they could do a better job reaching out to patients with hypothyroidism.

* * *

Indeed, there are clear signs that things are changing. In 2018 and 2019, Jacquie Jonklaas and her colleagues published a series of three surveys of physicians, members of the American Thyroid Association, about factors that affect therapy choice for hypothyroidism.[3]

Four hundred physicians were presented with different scenarios describing patients with hypothyroidism and were asked to choose between T_4 or combination therapy with T_4 and T_3. For patients without symptoms while on T_4, only 2% of the doctors would offer combination therapy. But if the patient had symptoms, that number increased to about 20%, whereas another 20% would simply increase the dose of T_4. If patients requested the addition of T_3 to their regimen, up to 35% of the doctors would prescribe it, and if the patient reported a previous positive experience with T_3, that number increased to 40%. Older age and the presence of osteoporosis reduced the number of physicians willing to prescribe combination therapy with T_4 and T_3.

* * *

I think we passed the point of no return in the fall of 2019 during the transatlantic live symposium in Chicago and London, sponsored by the American, British, and European Thyroid Associations. Experts from the United States and Europe presented their views and results on the treatment of hypothyroidism, with special emphasis on combination therapy. It was a cold Sunday morning in Chicago, but the room at the downtown Sheraton was packed. During the following year, we prepared and published a summary document, which served to update current clinical guidelines.[4]

The major achievement of this symposium was the recognition that the available trials comparing T_4 with combination therapy lack statistical power to address the issue of residual symptoms while on T_4. This is because most studies did not enroll sufficient numbers of patients who had residual symptoms. Several clinical trials have included subpopulations of patients who have symptoms at baseline while on T_4, but the small number of patients enrolled did not enable those trials to demonstrate clear benefit.

In other words, if we agree that only a minority of the patients with hypothyroidism do not feel well on T_4, then we should preferentially enroll those symptomatic patients in clinical trials that are testing therapy with T_4 and T_3. We need to enrich our study population with patients who did not benefit fully from T_4. Why include patients who feel well in these trials? If you feel well on T_4, you don't have a problem. It is unlikely that you will feel even better on combination therapy.

It is deeply disappointing that it took us fifty years to figure this out. The inclusion of patients who do well on T_4 in past clinical trials had the effect of diluting the effects of combination therapy on patients who remained symptomatic, decreasing the statistical power of the studies.

To appreciate this interference, imagine the following hypothetical scenario. An investigator wishes to study the effects of a new nutritional supplement to prevent breast cancer and figures he needs a thousand patients randomized into two groups. One group will receive a placebo and the other group will receive the new nutritional supplement. Patients will undergo screening for breast cancer annually for five years. Well, that plan is fine and the trial goes on, except that during recruitment, enrollment includes eight hundred men and two hundred women. And after randomization, the women are split about a hundred in each group.

The incidence of breast cancer in men is so small that their presence in the trial will mask whatever beneficial effect the new nutritional supplement might have. Such an enrollment pattern will decrease our ability to detect effects when we analyze the thousand individuals altogether. Believe it or not, this is exactly what we did in the last twenty trials or so that compared treatment with T_4 versus $T_4 + T_3$.

Therefore, it is expected that future trials will consider the recruitment of a sufficient number of individuals that exhibit residual symptoms on T_4, and patients are screened for genetic, autoimmune, and other interfering variables.

*　*　*

Based on everything discussed so far, today I am strongly inclined to offer a trial of therapy with $T_4 + T_3$ to most patients with hypothyroidism who remain symptomatic despite treatment with T_4. It is logical. It makes sense. Not only that. We now have data to back it up.

Yes, a few years ago I got to know Navy Captain Thanh D. Hoang, an endocrinologist working at the Walter Reed National Military Medical Center in Bethesda. Captain Hoang was born in Saigon and came to the United States as a teenager. He spent time at the NIH during high school and, upon becoming a doctor, joined the navy and trained just across the street, at Walter Reed Medical Center. He has always had a busy clinic, seeing about five hundred patients with hypothyroidism a year. He soon realized the current therapy is far from perfect.

He and his former mentor, Mohamed Shakir, designed a prospective, double-blind, crossover study with ninety patients with hypothyroidism randomly allocated to one of three four-month treatment groups: T_4, $T_4 + T_3$, or thyroid extract. At the end of each four months, the patients were evaluated and switched to a new therapy for four more months. A key point was to adjust the doses of the medications so that TSH levels would remain within normal range, independently of the treatment group. This would allow for a fair comparison across the treatment groups.[5]

While the study was in progress, Hoang and Shakir asked me to collaborate, and I gladly accepted. Seventy-five patients completed the study. While TSH levels did remain within reference range across all treatment groups, they observed the expected elevation in T_3 levels and reduction in T_4 levels when patients were on either form of combination therapy ($T_4 + T_3$ or thyroid extract). In line with previous clinical trials, there were no differences in quality of life, mood, cognition, and propensity for depression among the three treatment arms![6]

Having been part of the group that stressed the importance of focusing on T_4-treated symptomatic patients, I suggested we redirect our analysis to these patients. This was not straightforward because, to minimize bias, you can't just design a new data-analysis plan after the trial is completed and you see the results. To avoid bias, the investigator must create an analysis plan *before* the trial is started, which is registered at ClinicalTrials.gov and approved by the Institutional Review Board. If Hoang and Shakir wanted the focus to be on symptomatic patients, they should have spelled this out at the onset of the trial.

Daniel Brooks is a highly capable statistician at Walter Reed. Given the possibility of bias as described above, Brooks agreed to reanalyze the data as part of what is called an exploratory analysis. In this process, he broke down the study population into three similar-size groups of patients, according to their scores while they were on T_4. He teased out which patients performed poorly and were symptomatic on T_4. To simplify things, he used the scores to rank the patients as "very good," "good," and "poor" while on T_4.

The one-third of the patients who did "very good" on the tests were not symptomatic at all. They were fine on T_4, and after they switched to combination therapy, nothing happened. Their symptom scores remained low (the lower the score, the fewer the symptoms), similar to when they were on T_4.

Patients in the next third, the group that did "good," were slightly more symptomatic than the top performers, but were still fine on T_4, and exhibited no response to combination therapy.

However, the bottom third of patients, the ones who performed poorly, concentrated the patients who were symptomatic on T_4. They had the highest symptom scores and lowest quality of life while on T_4.

Anxiously, we waited for Brooks to finish up the analysis. We then looked at the scores after the patients were switched to combination therapy. They had improved markedly! These patients responded promptly to either form of combination therapy by minimizing their residual quality-of-life and cognitive symptoms, with either T_4 and T_3 or thyroid extract. Furthermore, the preference analysis indicated that this group showed a strong preference for combination therapy.

These were remarkable findings, especially because this was a relatively long double-blind crossover trial. The study confirmed that only some patients on T_4 therapy remain symptomatic despite normal serum TSH levels. And these are the ones who respond positively to and prefer either form of combination therapy.

As predicted by the combined American, British, and European task forces, these were the minority of the patients, and their outcome was not sufficient to affect the behavior of the whole group. However, in the subset analysis, these patients were identified as having the worst performance while on T_4, preferring and responding well to combination therapy. No issues with safety were identified. These findings suggest that thyroid-hormone action in a minority of the patients on T_4 remains subnormal and can be improved (perhaps restored) with the addition of T_3 to the therapy, to the benefit of the patient.

* * *

It has been a long journey, but we should continue with the clinical trials. We need to test all the variables involved, including age, sex, and genetic makeup. We also need to extend the safety record of the regimen using T_4 + T_3, particularly with older adults. Nonetheless, we must waste no time with hypothetical scenarios of concern and be more liberal in attempting combination therapy to those symptomatic patients. The patients have been waiting for too long.

Patients newly diagnosed with hypothyroidism should be treated with T_4. Most patients will do just fine. As we know, persistent symptoms are not uncommon and should prompt an investigation of other conditions that may present with similar symptoms. If nothing is identified and it seems uncontroverted that the patient has hypothyroidism and is not benefiting fully from therapy with T_4, a trial of combination therapy with T_4 + T_3 should be discussed with the patient.

Placing someone on combination therapy should be done thoughtfully. For the time being, I would not start anyone who has a cardiac condition without consultation from a cardiologist. Likewise, children and pregnant women should avoid combination therapy. Patients should be clear on what to expect: mainly, that it works for only some of the patients who remain symptomatic on T_4.

At this point, my preference is to initiate combination therapy with a tablet of levothyroxine (T_4) and a tablet of liothyronine (T_3), as opposed to thyroid extract. Using two separate tablets gives me the ability to adjust the dose of each hormone while monitoring two important and equally critical things: residual symptoms and TSH levels. We want to minimize residual symptoms while maintaining TSH within normal range. Using two separate medicines gives me flexibility in case I decide to prescribe a second replacement dose in the afternoon or at night. I want to do this with T_3 and not necessarily with the combination of T_4 and T_3 as in the thyroid extract.

Placing a patient on combination therapy requires an enhanced follow-up. Patients who are stable on T_4 can be seen every six months or once per year. I like to see patients on combination therapy more often than I see those on T_4 and to perform thyroid function tests and a careful clinical history to check for the occurrence of adverse reactions such as palpitations, anxiety, or a fine tremor. If needed, additional tests could be run. Common sense is critical here.

* * *

How is this done? Wilmar Wiersinga, the clinician-scientist at the University of Amsterdam, published an amazingly helpful template of how to initiate patients on combination therapy.[7] Based on his extensive clinical experience, this is a summary of what he recommends for patients who are on T_4 and wish to change to combination therapy with T_4 and T_3.

- If you are taking 100 micrograms of T_4 daily, switch to 87.5 micrograms of T_4 and 5 micrograms of T_3 daily.
- If you are taking 150 micrograms of T_4 daily, switch to 125 mcg of T_4 and 7.5 micrograms of T_3 daily.

- If you are on a dose of 200 micrograms of T_4 daily, switch to 175 micrograms of T_4 and 10 micrograms of T_3 daily.
- Other doses can be easily calculated based on these three references.

For all regimens, the daily T_3 dose should be divided—if possible—into two doses. The rationale is that the fast-moving T_3 peaks at about three hours after each dose. If you are splitting, Wiersinga recommends taking one dose before breakfast and the other dose before sleeping. If the amounts of the two doses are different (for example, 2.5 micrograms and 5 micrograms), the largest dose should be at night. This is because T_3 levels in the blood exhibit normal circadian rhythmicity with a peak at 4 a.m. and a valley at around 4 p.m. Alternatively, I recommend my patients take the second dose one hour before dinner. There is no magic formula. You and your doctor need to work together to see what suits you better. If, at any moment during treatment, measuring T_3 levels is needed, blood samples should be obtained twice: (1) while you are fasting in the morning and (2) about three hours after you take a T_3 tablet.

From a safety standpoint, it is reassuring to look at the analysis done by B. Van Tassell and colleagues, which included Francesco Celi. They calculated that for patients on T_4 + T_3 therapy, the addition of 2.5 to 10 micrograms of T_3 twice a day to their regimen is unlikely to result in spikes of circulating T_3 outside the normal reference range.[8]

The regimens described above should be considered as a starting point. Thus, minor adjustments will need to be made on a case-by-case basis. But which parameter should we use? Is it reasonable to optimize thyroid replacement based only or primarily on symptoms, or are thyroid function tests also helpful, even necessary? I believe both are important; but, with rare exceptions, the goal should be to use T_4 + T_3 to optimize symptoms without lowering TSH levels below normal range. In other words, we want to resolve symptoms while keeping the TSH levels within normal range. This is done by slightly lowering the T_4 dose and increasing the T_3 dose, followed by a new clinical assessment and TSH levels.

The outcome of a trial with combination therapy is unpredictable. It depends on the pool of patients that are seen by a specific physician. Endocrinologists tend to see the most complicated cases, so I bet that in their experience, combination therapy is more effective than as observed by primary care physicians—a Danish study revealed that 65% of patients with residual symptoms while on T_4 responded positively to this approach after twelve months.[9]

The ones who do respond invariably call or send me emails. Below is an example of a young man who reached out to me in the summer of 2019, when he was just about to start law school. His is not an unusual story[10] but some elements are key: he is a young man—no issues with menopause—and the residual symptoms can be traced back to the surgical thyroidectomy and treatment with T_4. He later sent me a follow-up message.

> The combination treatment didn't completely resolve the issues I have experienced but has definitely eased them. The biggest improvements have been in memory and in energy level. I have particularly noticed it in my energy level to take on additional responsibility (at school and at home) and have had the energy to stay significantly more organized. I have also noticed that I don't often feel like I am having difficulty remembering things.

> Conversations are much easier because I don't find myself forgetting what was just said which I often did before. Overall, with the combination treatment, I have had a much steadier day-to-day quality of life. I can say with confidence that this is the best I have felt in around 6 years since my thyroid originally started causing

me problems. Thank you so much for taking the time to sit down and talk with me, and for your thoughtful recommendation as it has made a tremendous impact in my life.

* * *

If you think you have residual symptoms despite treatment with T_4, you need to take action. Many patients with residual symptoms respond well to combination therapy *with the pharmaceuticals available today*. At the moment, we do have the means to improve patients' lives—many patients, millions of patients.

Start by educating yourself, discussing the issue with your family, and talking to your doctor. If you work, prepare yourself for the possibility that your performance will decline. Too many times I have seen family members in my office as frustrated as my patients, not understanding what was going on. As they understand your condition, they are the ones likely to give you the highest level of support. Alert your family and closest friends that your condition is likely to affect the way you interact with them. You might seem tired, unmotivated, spacy, forgetful. Remember, you are not alone. Recall my two patients in Miami and the hundreds more who answered the survey on brain fog. Mental work might seem particularly difficult until you find the resolution of your symptoms. Lower the expectations around your productivity for some time, and try not to take on major new tasks if you can.

Your doctor is the one who will be able to help you the most. A good relationship with your doctor is key for you getting better, maybe more so than with other thyroid conditions. Many patients like you find that their doctors are outstanding but do not have the time or availability to listen to them. This has been happening more and more because of the pressure placed by medical organizations on doctors. Even in good places, they want doctors to see a new patient every fifteen to twenty minutes. If you find that this is the case with your doctor, then you should look for another doctor, one who is used to cases such as yours, who understands the most recent clinical guidelines, and who has the time and is willing to help. Based on our survey results, you will feel better knowing that your doctor believes what you are saying and takes the time to listen to you.

Go online and look at physicians recommended by professional medical societies in your area. Call or email ahead explaining what you are looking for. Treatment is unlikely to involve very frequent visits, thus it is worth pursuing a doctor who you think is right for you, even if the office is not close to your home. Telemedicine has evolved rapidly in the last few years, so you could use this approach as well.

Once you get to the doctor, a good first step is to craft a plan to get you better. Set educated expectations and milestones. Together with your doctor, you should make sure you do have hypothyroidism. Of course, if you've had thyroid surgery or treatment with radioactive iodine, this is less likely to be a question. However, it could be an issue if you've been diagnosed with Hashimoto's disease.

Make sure to bring to the doctor old medical records that include TSH levels obtained at the time of your diagnosis. Tests showing that you tested positive for thyroperoxidase antibodies are also important. Online medical record systems have resolved many retrieval issues, but if you were diagnosed with hypothyroidism many years ago, you might need to call other offices to get old results. If you do not have access to old records, your doctor might ask you to stop treatment with T_4 for a couple of weeks and have your TSH levels measured. If you have hypothyroidism, TSH levels will increase above normal range. A thyroid ultrasound might help in some cases, as it may show a "patchy" pattern that is typical in patients with Hashimoto's disease.

Next, you and your doctor need to exclude associated conditions that could explain or worsen residual symptoms. In my experience, menopausal symptoms can mimic and/or exaggerate residual symptoms of hypothyroidism. But other conditions can too, particularly other autoimmune diseases. This step might require additional laboratory tests, so please be patient—it is worth getting a full picture of what is going on.

If, after going through these steps, nothing new is found, then you should discuss combination therapy with your doctor. That is the only thing we physicians can offer at this time that has some basis in science. If you go this route, your doctor will reduce your daily dose of T_4 and add T_3 to your daily regimen. Again, there is no predefined magic formula. It is really up to your doctor and their experience with this treatment.

Combination therapy could require a follow-up visit every three to four months, and a small number of additional tests. This is to ensure you remain safe throughout the treatment. You will know within a few weeks or a couple of months if this regimen works for you, though it could take longer. Adjustments in the doses of T_4 and T_3 could be tested at six-week intervals—this is the time the thyroid system takes to equilibrate into a new steady state. To be on the safe side, it is important to keep your TSH levels within normal range. This will ensure that you are not taking an excessive dose of thyroid hormones.

In my experience and that of my colleagues, about half the patients with residual symptoms will respond to combination therapy. Unfortunately, the other half will remain symptomatic. Thus, if after several adjustments you still do not see an improvement, then you should stop and resume treatment with T_4 only.

In this case, you and your doctors could again look for possible associated conditions that were not evident before. You could also try complementary approaches, which are not based on evidence-based medicine but anecdotally have helped patients with similar symptoms. In our survey about brain fog, patients felt better after resting, or by keeping a healthy diet; other patients improved after exercise.

Above all, try to draw strength from your supportive network of family and friends. Keep a positive attitude, because we still have a lot to learn about the thyroid gland. Promising new developments are in the pipeline. New ways of delivering T_3 are being developed, and several clinical trials focusing on symptomatic T_4-treated patients are on the way now. Soon we will have a much better understanding of your condition and an enhanced arsenal of medicines to help. This is discussed in the next chapter.

CHAPTER 15

The Promising Future

Given the historical concern with the fluctuation of circulating T_3 in patients treated with T_3, the 2014 American Thyroid Association guidelines recommend the development of new T_3 formulations with extended release that steadily restore T_3 levels to the normal reference range, without spikes.[1] For some of us, this has been the holy grail of treatment of hypothyroidism. Lew Braverman, the man who discovered T_4-to-T_3 conversion in humans and set off the shift from thyroid extract to monotherapy with T_4, wrote with Roti and colleagues in 1993 that perhaps the truly ideal therapy for hypothyroidism is T_4 + T_3 in a form in which the T_3 is slowly absorbed in a time-released fashion.[2]

A common strategy to delay the absorption of any drug is to use specially formulated tablets in which the drug is mixed with an excipient (filler), which delays the release of the drug into the intestine.[3] Scientists have tested multiple types of fillers and have even received patents for these methods. Unfortunately, when studied in patients, the desired "slow-release" isn't yet achieved (I can think of at least three major efforts that failed when tested clinically). In the early 2000s, Georg Hennemann and his colleagues reported some success with a specially prepared tablet formulation of T_3,[4] but he did not follow up with additional studies after the first one was published.

Nonetheless, in recent years, Ferruccio Santini, a clinician-scientist at the University of Pisa who had trained with Aldo Pinchera, a physician-scientist also in Pisa, has developed an ingenious strategy to achieve steady delivery of T_3. The new technology uses tablets containing a modified T_3 molecule (T_3-sulfate, a.k.a. T_3S). T_3S is inactive, but after meeting bacteria in patients' guts or passing through patients' livers, it is transformed into a fully active T_3 molecule that is returned to the circulation, identical to the T_3 produced by the body. Santini and his colleagues tested the hypothesis that T_3S might be used to treat hypothyroidism in rats and humans, with very promising results.[5]

Today, Santini sees about three hundred patients with hypothyroidism per year in his clinic in Pisa. He believes, as do many of us, that T_4 is sufficient to restore thyroid-hormone action in most patients with hypothyroidism, but it is not perfect. Santini believes that patients would be better served if we were also able to replace the small amounts of T_3 that are continuously secreted by the thyroid, normalizing the T_4:T_3 ratio in the circulation. But he is concerned that while administration of T_3 may produce apparent relief of some of the patients' complaints, it could also be associated with adverse reactions (mainly cardiac effects) that may pose risks, especially to older adult patients. His limited experience with T_3S showed patients' acceptance without evident signs of adverse reactions; unfortunately, though, he doesn't know if and when T_3S will be fully developed and commercially available for patients with hypothyroidism.

An interesting aspect of these studies was the involvement of Lew Braverman, the man who discovered T_4-to-T_3 conversion in humans. Braverman and Pinchera were very good friends. When Pinchera told him about their results with T_3S, he became enthusiastic about the project. After all, he was well aware of the limitations of T_4 monotherapy. Braverman was so excited about the project that he flew to Italy to discuss with an Italian pharmaceutical company the potential of T_3S in the treatment of hypothyroidism.

* * *

Thinking about novel T_3 supplementation strategies, for years I have concluded my lectures with a slide stating that pharmaceutical companies need to develop an improved delivery system for T_3, one that could avoid the spikes in T_3 levels and could therefore be used more broadly by patients with hypothyroidism, without safety concerns. Around 2015, I had just finished a lecture at Rush Hospital in Chicago when Scott Palmer, an internist there, approached me and mentioned he was part of a small startup that developed technology that could solve the problem of T_3 spikes after a T_3 tablet.

We had coffee, and I agreed to look at their technology purely on a scientific basis. I wanted to test the molecule in my laboratory with my resources and on my terms, without any external interference. I told them to let me first see the results. If it looked promising, we would talk further. I remember being asked what kind of statistical analysis I was planning on using, to which I replied, "None. If this drug works and is worth our time and effort, the results should be crystal clear and no statistics will be necessary."

In a few months, Tom Piccariello, the company's leading scientist, had created T_3 polymers complexed with different metals, of which zinc (poly-zinc-T_3, a.k.a. PZL) seemed the most promising, given the fact that zinc is already used in other drugs such as insulin and this widespread use is a testament to its safety. The mechanism of the extended release is that after a PZL capsule is swallowed, it travels through the stomach and dissolves in the intestine, where PZL is released and adheres to the intestinal walls. This creates an intestinal "drug depot" from which PZL is broken down and T_3 is gradually released and ultimately absorbed into the bloodstream.

I was ready to test the new molecule. I spoke to my fellows and they developed a system in which blood could be drawn multiple times from the tail vein of a rat during a period of twenty-four hours. The company delivered the capsules just days before each experiment. We were all blinded to the contents of each capsule, which were labeled A and B.

We did not know what to expect but, when the T_3 results came back, we immediately knew what was going on. Rats receiving the A capsules exhibited a slower elevation of T_3 in the circulation. No spikes were observed—just a smooth elevation in T_3 levels. After eight days of repeated administration of A capsules, steady T_3 levels were obtained.[6]

In contrast, the rats that received the B capsules exhibited a sharp spike in circulating-T_3 levels. TSH levels, which were elevated at the beginning of the experiment, declined rapidly after the B capsule, but in rats receiving the A capsules, the decline was delayed by about four hours.[7]

It was clear that the A capsules contained PZL and the B capsules contained regular T_3. PZL and T_3 had similar long-term biological effects, such as reduction of cholesterol levels, restoration of growth rate, and effects in the heart, liver, and brain—only, PZL did it without T_3 peaks in the circulation. This indicates that despite the slower absorption, PZL can have similar physiological effects as T_3.[8]

* * *

These experiments were repeated several times, with different doses of PZL and T_3. The results were confirmed each time. I agreed to assist further in the development of this new drug. There is so much excitement with PZL that in 2019 the National

Institutes of Health awarded the company and the University of Chicago with a grant to develop PZL for clinical trials in humans. The company synthesized PZL using standards of Current Good Manufacturing Practice and passed preclinical toxicological studies in rats and dogs. They next filed an exploratory Investigational New Drug (IND) application with the FDA, which was granted, and the University of Chicago's Institutional Review Board (IRB) approved the first clinical trial.

Alexandra Dumitrescu, my colleague in the Section of Endocrinology, agreed to serve as the principal investigator of the studies. She has experience with studies involving T_3 administration. I had no idea how much work was involved. The trial called for forty-eight-hour admission of twelve volunteers to the Clinical Research Center of the university. This was to be a double-blind, placebo-controlled crossover study. That means everyone was admitted three times with a two-week washout period in between admissions. Every little detail had to be well thought out and spelled out in many documents.

Recruitment wasn't smooth. People often have concerns about being "guinea pigs" when new drugs need to be tested. Despite confidence in getting enough volunteers, it was not easy. The recruiters had to advertise across all medical campuses in Chicago and make several phone calls. Finally, enrollment was completed, and the company finalized the preparation of the PZL capsules on time. They were delivered to the University of Chicago Research Pharmacy, where they were stored.

On the day of the trial, February 15, 2021, a record-breaking snowstorm hit Chicago. Nurses were waiting at the university, but cars could not move and there was no public transportation. I was home, but they asked me to drive by the homes of the volunteers and bring as many as I could to the university. We were a couple of hours late, but they were admitted, and the trial started as planned. Baseline blood samples were collected; one hour later, volunteers were ready to swallow the capsules with unknown contents (it could be T_3, PZL, or a placebo). They all stayed in individual rooms for the next forty-eight hours, and blood samples were obtained periodically for measurements of TSH, T_4, and T_3.

The results were very encouraging. When the volunteers took T_3, the expected peak of T_3 in the circulation developed two to three hours later. However, taking PZL caused T_3 levels to rise slowly and to a lower plateau that lasted about six hours. At no time during the first twenty-four hours did the T_3 levels drop below 50% of the peak in those patients who took PZL.[9]

The company is now working on their drug product development, wrapping up the last details of how the new drug will be packaged in a capsule. The final product will be tested one more time, and the results resubmitted to the FDA for approval.

* * *

Several new strategies and compounds to deliver a steady supply of T_3 to the circulation are being explored by many companies, but details aren't always available, due to commercial interests and the protection of intellectual property. These include liquid formulations (drops of a T_3 solution to be taken by mouth), chewable gums containing T_3, a subcutaneous implant of a gel or pellet that slowly releases T_3, hybrid molecules containing T_3, and T_3-containing nanoparticles.

To my knowledge, the most unusual approach is the use of a thermal inkjet printer that deposits T_3 onto a special paper. Little paper dots can be cut or detached and placed in the mouth, where it disintegrates in less than forty-five seconds. Studies in humans have not been performed yet, but the prospect of fine customization of T_3 dosages at home is very exciting.

Inspired by the success of the application of estrogen and testosterone on the patient's skin, some scientists considered developing a T_3 cream or patch that could be used by hypothyroid patients. It did not work. It turns out the skin metabolizes thyroid hormones at a very fast pace. Studies done in Pisa, by Ferruccio Santini and Aldo Pinchera and their colleagues, demonstrated that only about 20% of what is applied to the skin ever reaches circulation.[10] This remains a possible route if and when we can figure out how to protect the thyroid hormones from being inactivated in the skin.

*   *   *

So far, T_3S and PZL have shown promising results in animal and human studies. There is no doubt that the momentum around developing new delivery methods of T_3 for humans is building. This will pave the road to better understand and evaluate the use of combination therapy and possibly improve the lives of patients with hypothyroidism.

But I have left perhaps the most exciting development for last. I believe Tom Scanlan, an amazing organic chemist at Oregon Health & Science University, is in many ways on track to change the way we think about thyroid-hormone supplementation. He is certainly at the level of the discipline-changing figures we have already discussed—Edward Kendall, Charles Harington, and Rosalind Pitt-Rivers. He used the information obtained from the crystallization of the thyroid-hormone receptor to develop new molecules that "look like" T_3, but that do not have iodine in their structure.

One of these molecules is sobetirome, which can initiate thyroid-hormone action in selective organs. For example, sobetirome mimics the effects of thyroid hormones in the liver, adipose tissue, and brain, without affecting the heart or the bones. This is mind boggling. But that is not all. Tom had an even more daring idea. He created an inherently inactive prodrug of sobetirome that can only be activated once it reaches the inside of the brain! So, he showed in mice that this drug can treat brain hypothyroidism while only minimally affecting the other organs in the body.

Some of these drugs have been tested in clinical trials while for others the trials are currently underway. It is not an overstatement to say that these new molecules have the potential to revolutionize the treatment of hypothyroidism. You can follow their progress and that of any other drug at ClinicalTrials.gov.

*   *   *

As we saw, a thyroid gland transplant was the first reasonably successful approach to treat hypothyroidism. Despite early successes, thyroid transplant was abandoned because the graft did not take and symptoms kept recurring. More recently, Sabine Costagliola, a scientist at the Institut de Recherche Interdisciplinaire en Biologie Humaine et Moléculaire in Bruxelles, Belgium, collaborated with Sam Refetoff and Alexandra Dumitrescu at the University of Chicago, and developed a method to generate new thyroid cells from the stem (progenitor) cells.[11] After these thyroid cells were grafted near the kidney of a mouse with hypothyroidism, they organized as if in a normal thyroid gland, restoring thyroid-hormone levels in the mouse!

Other groups in the United States have reproduced and expanded these experiments[12] and, as a whole, it is now clear that thyroid-hormone levels can be restored to normal in mice with hypothyroidism by transplanting thyroid organoids derived from stem cells. More recently, Terry Davies, a physician-scientist at Mount Sinai Hospital in New York, and his colleagues used stem cells (that were differentiated to be thyroid cells) to restore thyroid-hormone levels in a severely hypothyroid mouse for almost six months.[13]

This technology is moving fast. The next logical step already achieved in a few laboratories is to use human cells. Thanks to Shinya Yamanaka's lab in Kyoto, human stem cells obtained from the skin can be engineered in the laboratory to develop into any other cell of your body. Once developed, they can be transferred back to your body. For his discovery, he was awarded the 2012 Nobel Prize in Physiology or Medicine along with John Gurdon. Since these stem cells are derived directly from adult organs, they not only bypass the need for embryos but can be made in a patient-matched manner, which means that each individual could have their own stem-cell line.

Scientists in the thyroid field took cells from the skin of a donor (fibroblasts) and made them into human stem cells that subsequently formed functional thyroid cells. This is amazing! It lays the groundwork for future person-specific thyroid regenerative therapy. I remain positive that this will prove feasible in humans. Patients complaining of persistent hypothyroidism symptoms could benefit from a new thyroid gland and physiological secretion of both T_3 and T_4.

EPILOGUE

For years I reflected on how to organize a book that captured what has happened and is now happening in the world of hypothyroidism. What went so wrong to have us fail to consider those patients who remained symptomatic on T_4? I talk about this with colleagues, friends, and family members, trying to figure out, to make sense of what has happened during the last fifty years. It was my brother, João, who said, "Sometimes we can't see what's right in front of us."

Psychologists talk about such mental blind spots. In medicine, we call a blind spot a scotoma. In psychology, the term originally used by the French neurologist Jean-Martin Charcot was reintroduced in the 1920s by the two French psychoanalysts René Laforgue and Edouard Pinchon. A "psychological scotoma" means that we have information gained from previous experiences that we repress or ignore, and we end up turning a blind eye to those things. We do this because of preconceived beliefs. They may make us fail to see a solution just because it doesn't fit in nicely with our current thinking and worldview.

It is fascinating that the Scottish physician William W. Ireland wrote in 1900: "It looks now like a strange blindness that physicians were so long in seeing that the common cause of cretinism . . . and of myxedema, lay in the deficiency . . . of the thyroid gland. But pathologists were prevented from more speedily discerning this relation by confident statements that . . . there was no affection of the thyroid gland."[1]

In retrospect, it seems like more recently many physicians are still falling into a similar trap. We were well aware that new therapies must be tested and retested before we can recommend them to patients. Yet, our belief that T_4-to-T_3 conversion would resolve hypothyroidism and that TSH is the best possible way to adjust the dose of T_4 was so strong that, along with the regulatory loopholes at the FDA, we skipped those rigorous trials.

Deiodinases were at the core of these two beliefs, and this was so novel and fascinating that we wanted to believe they could do the job. The dogma led us to believe that treatment with T_4 would restore things to the way they were before hypothyroidism. And we were getting good feedback—most patients responded well to T_4. Not until decades later did some of us start asking ourselves how *all* patients feel on T_4—or simply what they prefer. It took much grief for us to open our eyes. Patients were embarrassed and ashamed by what they had become; they were losing their jobs, disrupting their families.

Things were right there in front of our eyes. Since 1970, some patients were already saying that they were not feeling well, that they were experiencing residual symptoms of hypothyroidism. They wrote letters, sent emails, and signed petitions. Yes, we knew from studies done in Cardiff, Amsterdam, and Portland that treatment with T_4 did not restore quality of life or cognition for all patients. We also knew that it did not restore T_3 levels— the molecule that we understood is the most important thyroid hormone.

However, most of the time, we just ignored the evidence, didn't talk about it. We set a bar for combination therapy that was so much higher than the one set for T_4 in the 1970s.

*　　*　　*

I feel the biggest consequence of our collective blind spot was to ignore patients who were (and still are) suffering. Not acknowledging these patients in our guidelines for what they are— namely, examples of T_4's failings—was not right. Not alerting physicians in our medical schools, lectures, courses, and clinical guidelines to be aware of the fact that 10–20% of the T_4-treated patients fail to fully recover from hypothyroidism was a mistake. We might not have had the answer, but continuing with the rosy T_4 scenario without asking the hard questions and facing the problem was plain wrong.

According to psychologists, one way to avoid a blind spot is to give the benefit of the doubt or step into someone's shoes. Those two patients in Miami impressed me so much. Without realizing it, I started looking at things from their perspective and became very skeptical of the dogmas that, until then, I had fully accepted and embraced. I pivoted my research, truly believing that things were not right and something needed to be done.

*　　*　　*

While I remain disappointed with the past, there is good reason to be excited about the future. Developments in the world of hypothyroidism over the last few years indicate that physicians and professional societies got the message and are moving in the right direction. More and more physicians are accepting that patients with hypothyroidism may exhibit residual symptoms despite treatment, and new data has become available that the long-term safety record of the current T_3 preparations. In addition, new strategies to administer T_3 are being developed by the pharmaceutical industry. I do see hope and optimism among my colleagues that things will improve.

More progress will depend on a few important steps. The message coming from professional medical organizations must change to officially recognize the existence of patients with residual symptoms while on T_4. They should make it crystal clear to their members and constituents that one or two in every ten patients with hypothyroidism on T_4 remain symptomatic and the symptoms are thyroid related. These patients exhibit a condition that should have a name—for example, syndrome of residual symptoms of hypothyroidism on T_4 (SORSHOT).

After being ignored for decades, these patients must be publicly acknowledged. The existence of SORSHOT needs to be officially recognized; perhaps an ICD number should be created. The FDA should require the makers of T_4 to disclose its limitations on the box label. This will alert physicians and signal to the patients that we hear them. It will help streamline funds from agencies and foundations that sponsor research in this area.

I also think that professional medical associations that prepared guidelines during these last fifty years owe to the patients an explanation. The fact that we ignored a portion of our patients for so long, despite evidence to the contrary, needs to be reckoned with if we are to regain credibility.

Medical associations should organize task forces to characterize the true SORSHOT. This would help physicians to identify patients with this syndrome. We need to know how to diagnose these patients, and how to distinguish SORSHOT patients from other symptomatic patients in whom hypothyroidism is well compensated on T_4.

The task forces should also develop algorithms that can easily be used by physicians whenever they are faced with a patient whom they suspect SORSHOT. These algorithms should start by having the physician acknowledge to the patient that we are aware that this syndrome exists and, although we are still learning how to diagnose and treat it, we will attempt modifications of the treatment to help the patient.

Education of physicians through CME courses about SOR-SHOT is very important. More emphasis should be given to the fact that T_3 can and should be safely tried in patients with the syndrome. The emphasis should be changed from complete avoidance, given limited safety data, to guidelines for use based on the data that exists. Education should also encompass the concept that a formal diagnosis of hypothyroidism is required before placing anyone on T_4. It is our responsibility to explain that only hypothyroid patients should be treated with thyroid hormones.

Federal funds need to be made available so that scientists can investigate the mechanistic basis for SORSHOT. There are likely a host of factors, including genetic predisposition, and associated diseases. Low T_3 levels most likely play a role, but the principles of evidence-based medicine require that more clinical evidence be obtained. What we have now is a logical conjecture, but abundant conclusive data is missing.

Following the most recent recommendations of the American, British, and European Thyroid Associations, clinical scientists should design trials that focus on patients who have SORSHOT to determine whether any old or new treatment provides symptom relief. More studies addressing the long-term safety of T_3 or thyroid extract are also needed.

ACKNOWLEDGMENTS

I am grateful to several individuals without whom this book would not be possible. My wonderful parents, Elide and Mario Bianco, for everything. My fellows and students, as I have been fortunate to have had the best summer students, undergrads, grad students, and postdoctoral fellows, many of whom are featured in the book. My patients, from whom I learned much of what was discussed in this book. My scientific collaborators, who graciously shared reagents and animals, and agreed to collaborate on so many projects. John Harney, an exceptional human being from whom I learned so much. Joseph Calamia, for his outstanding and tireless editorial work, Johanna Rosenbohm and Lindsy Rice, for the superb copyediting work, and Amanda Moon, for assisting me with the vision of the book. Marla Berry, Colin Dayan, Val Galton, Colum Gorman, Damiano Gullo, Thanh Hoang, David Ingbar, Jacquie Jonklaas, Peter Kopp, Rui M. B. Maciel, John Morris, Amanda Pearl, Mary Samuels, Ferruccio Santini, J. Enrique Silva, Martin Surks, Peter Taylor, Connie Trump, Wilmar Wiersinga, Graham Williams, and Marvin Wool for providing details of their work, their lives, and suggesting additional sources for my research. My wife, Miriam Ribeiro, and children, Laura Bianco, George Bianco, and Michael Bianco, my brothers João F. Bianco and Salvador M. Bianco, and my colleagues Samuel Refetoff and Brian Kim for critically reading and commenting on different parts of the manuscript while the work was in progress. To the Mayo Foundation for Medical Education and Research, courtesy of the W. Bruce Fye Center for the History of Medicine, Mayo Clinic, and kind and professional staff, for allowing me to research their archives.

Lastly, I am a consultant for AbbVie, the maker of Synthroid and Armour Thyroid; for Synthonics, the maker of PZL; and for Thyron, which is developing new technology to modulate thyroid-hormone action. I have occasionally consulted for IBSA, the maker of Thyrosint. My immediate family and I own no stocks or stock options in any of these companies and have not received research grants from pharmaceutical companies or been involved in promotional activities of pharmaceutical products.

NOTES

CHAPTER 1

1. J. H. Means, L. J. DeGroot, J. B. Stanbury, "Adult Hypothyroid States," in *The Thyroid and Its Diseases*, ed. Means, DeGroot, and Stanbury (New York: McGraw-Hill, 1963), 329.

2. S. Taylor, M. Kapur, and R. Adie, "Combined Thyroxine and Triiodothyronine for Thyroid Replacement Therapy," *British Medical Journal* 2, no. 5704 (1970): 270–71.

3. N. D. Roberts, "Psychological Problems in Thyroid Disease," *British Thyroid Foundation Newsletter*, 1996.

4. See S. J. Peterson, A. R. Cappola, M. R. Castro, et al., "An Online Survey of Hypothyroid Patients Demonstrates Prominent Dissatisfaction," *Thyroid* 28, no. 6 (2018): 707–21.

5. Bitterinternist, "It's Not Your Thyroid," YouTube video, 3 minutes, 8 seconds, https://www.youtube.com/watch?v=zgL405Scrpa.

6. "Not a Conspiracy Theory: Our Campaign Tactics," Thyroid Patients Canada, April 22, 2019, https://thyroidpatients.ca/2019/04/22/not-a-conspiracy-theory-our-campaign-tactics/.

7. See J. P. Brito, J. S. Ross, O. M. El Kawkgi, et al., "Levothyroxine Use in the United States, 2008–2018," *JAMA Internal Medicine* 181 no. 10 (2021): 1402–5.

8. Peterson, Cappola, Castro, et al., "Online Survey of Hypothyroid Patients."

9. See A. C. Bianco and P. R. Larsen, "Tranquil Plasma Surrounding an Intracellular Storm," *Thyroid* 15, no. 8 (2005): 751.

10. See A. C. Bianco, S. Ribich, and B. W. Kim, "An Inside Job," *Endocrinology* 148, no. 7 (2007): 3077–79.

11. B. M. Bocco, R. A. Louzada, D. H. Silvestre, et al., "Thyroid Hormone Activation by Type 2 Deiodinase Mediates Exercise-Induced Peroxisome Proliferator-Activated Receptor-Gamma Coactivator-1alpha Expression in Skeletal Muscle," *Journal of Physiology* 594, no. 18 (2016): 5255–69.

12. L. E. Braverman, S. H. Ingbar, and K. Sterling, "Conversion of Thyroxine (T4)

to Triiodothyronine (T3) in Athyreotic Subjects," *Journal of Clinical Investigation* 49, no. 5 (1970): 855–64.

13. J. Jonklaas, A. C. Bianco, A. J. Bauer, et al., "Guidelines for the Treatment of Hypothyroidism: Prepared by the American Thyroid Association Task Force on Thyroid Hormone Replacement," *Thyroid* 24, no. 12 (2014): 1670–751.

CHAPTER 2

1. A. M. Tybout, J. Hennessy, N. Fahey, and C. Snyder, "The Case of Synthroid (A): Marketing a Drug Coming Off Patent," *Kellogg School of Management Cases* (2017): 1–19.

2. P. J. Hilts, "After 46 Years of Sales, Thyroid Drug Needs F.D.A. Approval," *New York Times*, July 24, 2001, section 1.

3. See Braverman, Ingbar, and Sterling, "Conversion of Thyroxine (T4) to Triiodothyronine (T3)."

4. See Tybout, Hennessy, Fahey, and Snyder, "The Case of Synthroid (A)"; and J. Hennessy, A. M. Tybout, N. Fahey, and C. Snyder, "The Case of Synthroid (B): Marketing a Drug Coming Off Patent," *Kellogg School of Management Cases* (2017): 1–8.

5. See Braverman, Ingbar, and Sterling, "Conversion of Thyroxine (T4) to Triiodothyronine (T3)."

6. Hennessy, Tybout, Fahey, and Snyder, "The Case of Synthroid (B)."

7. "Global Levothyroxine Market Outlook 2022," Absolute Reports, January 4, 2022, https://www.absolutereports.com/global-levothyroxine-market-19862496.

8. R. T. King, "How Drug Firm Paid for Study by University, Then Yanked It," *Wall Street Journal*, April 25, 1996.

9. P. Sherrod, "Baxter Completes Sale of Flint Labs," *Chicago Tribune*, September 4, 1986.

10. S. H. Curry, J. G. Gums, L. L. Williams, R. W. Curry, B. B. Wolfson, "Levothyroxine Sodium Tablets: Chemical Equivalence and Bioequivalence," *Drug Intelligence & Clinical Pharmacy* 22, nos. 7–8 (1988): 589–91.

11. King, "How Drug Firm Paid for Study." The following paragraphs are sourced from this article.

12. King. The following paragraphs are sourced from this article.

13. G. H. Mayor, T. Orlando, and N. M. Kurtz, "Limitations of Levothyroxine Bioequivalence Evaluation: Analysis of an Attempted Study," *American Journal of Therapeutics* 2, no. 6 (1995): 417–32, quotation on 417.

14. L. K. Altman, "Drug Firm, Relenting, Allows Unflattering Study to Appear," *New York Times*, April 16, 1997, sect. 1; B. J. Dong, W. W. Hauck, J. G. Gambertoglio, et al., "Bioequivalence of Generic and Brand-Name Levothyroxine Products in the Treatment of Hypothyroidism," *JAMA* 277, no. 15 (1997): 1205–13.

15. See D. Rennie, "Thyroid Storm," *JAMA* 277, no. 15 (1997): 1238–43.

16. C. H. Eckert, "Bioequivalence of Levothyroxine Preparations: Industry Sponsorship and Academic Freedom," *JAMA* 277, no. 15 (1997): 1200; Altman, "Drug Firm, Relenting, Allows Unflattering Study"; Hilts, "After 46 Years of Sales."

17. See Dong, Hauck, Gambertoglio, et al., "Bioequivalence of Generic and Brand-Name Levothyroxine Products"; and Braverman, Ingbar, and Sterling, "Conversion of Thyroxine (T4) to Triiodothyronine (T3)."

18. See C. Adams, "FDA Could Make Abbott Pull Synthroid, Popular Thyroid Drug, from the Market," *Wall Street Journal*, June 1, 2001; and Hilts, "After 46 Years of Sales."

19. "FDA Approves Synthroid, Clearing Hurdle for Abbott," *Wall Street Journal*, July 25, 2002.

20. Amanda Perl, executive director, American Thyroid Association, email message to author, October 25, 2021.

CHAPTER 3

1. W. L. Green, "Guidelines for the Treatment of Myxedema," *Medical Clinics of North America* 52, no. 2 (1968): 431–50.

2. See Braverman, Ingbar, and Sterling, "Conversion of Thyroxine (T4) to Triiodothyronine (T3)."

3. H. A. Selenkow and L. I. Rose, "Comparative Clinical Pharmacology of Thyroid Hormones," in *The Thyroid Physiology and Treatment of Disease*, ed. J. M. Hershman and G. A. Bray (Oxford: Pergamon Press, 1976), 331–49.

4. P. A. Singer, D. S. Cooper, E. G. Levy, et al., "Treatment Guidelines for Patients with Hyperthyroidism and Hypothyroidism: Standards of Care Committee, American Thyroid Association," *JAMA* 273, no. 10 (1995): 808–12.

5. Taylor, Kapur, and Adie, "Combined Thyroxine and Triiodothyronine," 270.

6. See J. M. Stock, M. I. Surks, and J. H. Oppenheimer, "Replacement Dosage of L-thyroxine in Hypothyroidism: A Re-evaluation," *New England Journal of Medicine* 290, no. 10 (1974): 529–33; J. C. Ingbar, M. Borges, S. Iflah, R. E. Kleinmann, L. E. Braverman, and S. H. Ingbar, "Elevated Serum Thyroxine Concentration in Patients Receiving 'Replacement' Doses of Levothyroxine," *Journal of Endocrinological Investigation* 5, no. 2 (1982): 77–85; E. C. Ridgway, D. S. Cooper, H. Walker, et al., "Therapy of Primary Hypothyroidism with L-triiodothyronine: Discordant Cardiac and Pituitary Responses," *Clinical Endocrinology* 13, no. 5 (1980): 479–88; P. E. Jennings, B. P. O'Malley, K. E. Griffin, B. Northover, and F. D. Rosenthal, "Relevance of Increased Serum Thyroxine Concentrations Associated with Normal Serum Triiodothyronine Values in Hypothyroid Patient Receiving Thyroxine: A Case for 'Tissue Thyrotoxicosis,'" *British Medical Journal* 289 (1984): 1645–47; C. J. Pearce and R. L. Himsworth, "Total and Free Thyroid Hormone Concentrations in Patients Receiving Maintenance Replacement Treatment with Thyroxine," *British Medical Journal (Clinical Research*

Edition) 288, no. 6418 (1984): 693–95; L. H. Fish, H. L. Schwartz, J. Cavanaugh, M. W. Steffes, J. P. Bantle, and J. H. Oppenheimer, "Replacement Dose, Metabolism, and Bioavailability of Levothyroxine in the Treatment of Hypothyroidism," *New England Journal of Medicine* 316 (1987): 764–70; A. Kahn, "Serum Triiodothyronine Levels in Patients Receiving L-thyroxine," *Clinical Pharmacology & Therapeutics* 19, no. 5 pt. 1 (1976): 523–30; L. E. Murchison, M. I. Chesters, and P. D. Bewsher, "Serum Thyroid Hormone Levels in Patients on Thyroxine Replacement Therapy," *Hormone and Metabolic Research* 8, no. 4 (1976): 324–25; D. Salmon, M. Rendell, J. Williams, et al., "Chemical Hyperthyroidism: Serum Triiodothyronine Levels in Clinically Euthyroid Individuals Treated with Levothyroxine," *Archives of Internal Medicine* 142, no. 3 (1982): 571–73; E. M. Erfurth and P. Hedner, "Thyroid Hormone Metabolism in Thyroid Disease as Reflected by the Ratio of Serum Triiodothyronine to Thyroxine," *Journal of Endocrinological Investigation* 9, no. 5 (1986): 407–12; and Taylor, Kapur, and Adie, "Combined Thyroxine and Triiodothyronine."

7. H. J. Baskin, R. H. Cobin, D. S. Duick, et al., "American Association of Clinical Endocrinologists Medical Guidelines for Clinical Practice for the Evaluation and Treatment of Hyperthyroidism and Hypothyroidism," *Endocrine Practice* 8, no. 6 (2002): 457–69.

8. Roberts, "Psychological Problems in Thyroid Disease."

9. J. R. Garber, R. H. Cobin, H. Gharib, et al., "Clinical Practice Guidelines for Hypothyroidism in Adults: Cosponsored by the American Association of Clinical Endocrinologists and the American Thyroid Association," *Thyroid* 22, no. 12 (2012): 1200–1235.

10. See P. Saravanan, W. F. Chau, N. Roberts, K. Vedhara, R. Greenwood, and C. M. Dayan, "Psychological Well-Being in Patients on 'Adequate' Doses of L-thyroxine: Results of a Large, Controlled Community-Based Questionnaire Study," *Clinical Endocrinology* 57, no. 5 (2002): 577–85; and E. M. Wekking, B. C. Appelhof, E. Fliers, et al., "Cognitive Functioning and Well-Being in Euthyroid Patients on Thyroxine Replacement Therapy for Primary Hypothyroidism," *European Journal of Endocrinology* 153, no. 6 (2005): 747–53.

11. K. Petersen, C. Bengtsson, L. Lapidus, G. Lindstedt, and E. Nystrom, "Morbidity, Mortality, and Quality of Life for Patients Treated with Levothyroxine," *Archives of Internal Medicine* 150, no. 10 (1990): 2077–81.

12. T. Idrees, S. Palmer, R. M. B. Maciel, and A. C. Bianco, "Liothyronine and Desiccated Thyroid Extract in the Treatment of Hypothyroidism," *Thyroid* 30, no. 10 (2020): 1399–413.

13. W. M. Wiersinga, L. Duntas, V. Fadeyev, B. Nygaard, and M. P. Vanderpump, "2012 ETA Guidelines: The Use of L-T4 + L-T3 in the Treatment of Hypothyroidism," *European Thyroid Journal* 1, no. 2 (2012): 55–71.

CHAPTER 4

1. S. Slater, "The Discovery of Thyroid Replacement Therapy: Part 1: In the Beginning," *Journal of the Royal Society of Medicine* 104, no. 1 (2011): 15–18. William Prout in London may have been the first to use iodine to treat goiter as early as 1816, five years after iodine was discovered. However, it seems he only treated one patient and did not publish until 1834, saying he was instrumental in St. Thomas' Hospital adopting the remedy in 1819.

2. W. W. Ireland, *Cretinism: The Mental Affections of Children* (Philadelphia: P. Blakiston's Son, 1900).

3. Ireland, *Cretinism*.

4. D. Marine, "Etiology and Prevention of Simple Goiter," *Medicine (Baltimore)* 3, no. 453 (1924): 453–66.

5. Slater, "Discovery of Thyroid Replacement Therapy: Part 1."

6. P. N. Taylor, D. Albrecht, A. Scholz, et al., "Global Epidemiology of Hyperthyroidism and Hypothyroidism," *Nature Reviews Endocrinology* 14, no. 5 (2018): 301–16.

7. A. C. Bianco, A. Dumitrescu, B. Gereben, et al., "Paradigms of Dynamic Control of Thyroid Hormone Signaling," *Endocrine Reviews* 40, no. 4 (2019): 1000–1047.

8. P. R. Larsen, J. E. Silva, and M. M. Kaplan, "Relationships between Circulating and Intracellular Thyroid Hormones: Physiological and Clinical Implications," *Endocrine Reviews* 2, no. 1 (1981): 87–102.

9. S. Jo, T. L. Fonseca, B. Bocco, et al., "Type 2 Deiodinase Polymorphism Causes ER Stress and Hypothyroidism in the Brain," *Journal of Clinical Investigation* 129, no. 1 (2019): 230–45; M. G. Castagna, M. Dentice, S. Cantara, et al., "DIO2 Thr92Ala Reduces Deiodinase-2 Activity and Serum-T3 Levels in Thyroid-Deficient Patients," *Journal of Clinical Endocrinology and Metabolism* 102, no. 5 (2017): 1623–30.

10. See M. M. Franca, A. German, G. W. Fernandes, et al., "Human Type 1 Iodothyronine Deiodinase (DIO1) Mutations Cause Abnormal Thyroid Hormone Metabolism," *Thyroid* 31, no. 2 (2021): 202–7.

CHAPTER 5

1. Larsen, Silva, and Kaplan, "Relationships between Circulating and Intracellular Thyroid Hormones."

2. The thyroid secretes T_3 into the circulation. At the same time, organs that have deiodinases also dump T_3 into the circulation. These organs take up T_4 and convert to T_3, which then leaves the organs and returns to the circulation. Thus, at all times, the T_3 in the circulation represents the mixture of T_3 secreted directly from the thyroid with the T_3 produced outside the thyroid gland via the deiodinases. This large pool of circulating T_3 is the source of T_3 that enters all organs and triggers biological effects.

3. A. C. Bianco and J. E. Silva, "Intracellular Conversion of Thyroxine to Triiodo-

thyronine Is Required for the Optimal Thermogenic Function of Brown Adipose Tissue," *Journal of Clinical Investigation* 79, no. 1 (1987): 295–300; A. C. Bianco and J. E. Silva, "Optimal Response of Key Enzymes and Uncoupling Protein to Cold in BAT Depends on Local T3 Generation," *American Journal of Physiology* 253, no. 3, part 1 (1987): E255–63; A. C. Bianco and J. E. Silva, "Nuclear 3,5,3'-triiodothyronine (T3) in Brown Adipose Tissue: Receptor Occupancy and Sources of T3 as Determined by *in vivo* Techniques," *Endocrinology* 120, no. 1 (1987): 55–62.

4. M. M. Baqui, B. Gereben, J. W. Harney, P. R. Larsen, and A. C. Bianco, "Distinct Subcellular Localization of Transiently Expressed Types 1 and 2 Iodothyronine Deiodinases as Determined by Immunofluorescence Confocal Microscopy," *Endocrinology* 141, no. 11 (2000): 4309–12.

5. V. A. Galton, P. R. Larsen, and M. J. Berry, "The Deiodinases: Their Identification and Cloning of Their Genes," *Endocrinology* 162, no. 3 (2021).

6. M. J. Berry and P. R. Larsen, "The Role of Selenium in Thyroid Hormone Action," *Endocrine Reviews* 13, no. 2 (1992): 207–19.

7. C. Curcio, M. M. Baqui, D. Salvatore, et al., "The Human Type 2 Iodothyronine Deiodinase Is a Selenoprotein Highly Expressed in a Mesothelioma Cell Line," *Journal of Biological Chemistry* 276, no. 32 (2001): 30183–87.

8. I. Callebaut, C. Curcio-Morelli, J. P. Mornon, et al., "The Iodothyronine Selenodeiodinases Are Thioredoxin-Fold Family Proteins Containing a Glycoside Hydrolase Clan GH-A-like Structure," *Journal of Biological Chemistry* 278, no. 38 (2003): 36887–96.

CHAPTER 6

1. See Honoré de Balzac, *The Country Doctor* (Philadelphia: George Barrie & Son, 1898).

2. Mark Twain, *A Tramp Abroad* (London: Chatto, 1880), 203.

3. *Rapport de la commission créée par S. M. le Roi de Sardaigne, pour étudier le cretinisme* (Turin: Imprimerie Royale, 1848).

4. The Royal London Hospital is a large teaching hospital in Whitechapel in the London Borough of Tower Hamlets. It is part of Barts Health NHS Trust. The Royal London provides district general hospital services for the City and Tower Hamlets and specialist tertiary care services for patients from across London and elsewhere.

5. T. B. Curling, "Two Cases of Absence of the Thyroid Body, and Symmetrical Swellings of Fat Tissue at the Sides of the Neck, Connected with Defective Cerebral Development," *Medico-Chirurgical Transactions* 33 (1850): 303–6.

6. Guy's Hospital is an NHS hospital in the borough of Southwark in Central London. It is part of Guy's and St. Thomas' NHS Foundation Trust and one of the institutions that is part of the King's Health Partners, an academic health science center.

7. C. H. Fagge, "On Sporadic Cretinism, Occurring in England," *Medico-Chirurgical Transactions* 54 (1871): 155–70.

8. Upon Gull's death in 1890, Mark Twain wrote, "Sir Wm. Gull is just dead. He nursed the Prince of Wales back to life in 1971 and apparently it was for this that Mr. Gull was granted a Knighthood, that doormat at the threshold of nobility. When the Prince seemed dead Mr. Gull dealt blow after blow between the shoulders, breathed into his nostrils, and literally cheated Death." A. B. Paine, ed., *Mark Twain's Notebook* (New York: Harper & Brothers, 1935), 209–10. And according to a 1970s conspiracy theory (widely dismissed by scholars), it was believed that Gull knew the identity of Jack the Ripper, or even that he was the murderer.

9. W. W. Gull, "On a Cretinoid State Supervening in Adult Life in Women," *Transactions of the Clinical Society of London* 7 (1874): 180–85.

10. Ord's career was interrupted in the late 1850s when circumstances compelled him to go into private practice to assist his father in Streatham, a suburb of London. Only in 1871 was he able to return to academics, after an opening on the medical staff allowed him to join as assistant physician. What followed was a meteoric career that led him to become the dean of the medical school.

11. St. Thomas' Hospital is a large NHS teaching hospital in Central London. It is one of the institutions of the King's Health Partners. Administratively part of the Guy's and St. Thomas' NHS Foundation Trust, together with Guy's Hospital, King's College Hospital, University Hospital Lewisham, and Queen Elizabeth Hospital, it provides the location of the King's College London GKT School of Medical Education. As one of London's oldest and most famous hospitals, it was named after St. Thomas Becket— which suggests it may have been founded after Becket's canonization in 1173. Today, Guy's and St. Thomas' Hospitals have merged, predestined to work together some three hundred years earlier when Thomas Guy, a governor of St. Thomas', founded Guy's Hospital as a place to treat "incurables" discharged from St. Thomas'.

12. W. M. Ord, "On Myxœdema, a Term Proposed to Be Applied to an Essential Condition in the 'Cretinoid' Affection Occasionally Observed in Middle-Aged Women," *Medico-Chirurgical Transactions* 61 (1878): 57–78.

13. J.-L. Reverdin, "Accidents consécutifs àl'ablation totale du goitre," *Reveu Médicale de la Suisse Romande* 2 (1882): 539–40.

14. P. Kopp, "Theodor Kocher (1841–1917), Nobel Prize Centenary 2009," *Arquivos brasileiros de endocrinologia e metabologia* 53, no. 9 (2009): 1176–80.

15. T. Kocher, "Ueber Kropfexstirpation und ihre Folgen," *Archiv für Klinische Chirurgie* 29 (1883): 254–337.

16. U. Tröhler, "Towards Endocrinology: Theodor Kocher's 1883 Account of the Unexpected Effects of Total Ablation of the Thyroid," *JLL Bulletin: Commentaries on the History of Treatment Evaluation*, 2010, https://www.jameslindlibrary.org/articles /towards-endocrinology-theodor-kochers-1883-account-of-the-unexpected-effects -of-total-ablation-of-the-thyroid/.

17. W. M. Ord, "Report of the Committee of the Clinical Society of London Nominated December 14, 1883, to Investigate the Subject of Myxoedema," *Transactions of*

the Clinical Society of London 21 (suppl.) (1888): 1–215. See also C. T. Sawin, "Defining Myxoedema and Its Cause," in *Report on Myxoedema* (Clinical Society of London, 1888; facsimile ed., 1991), 1–14.

18. E. T. Blake, "Myxedema," in *Myxœdema, Cretinism and the Goitres*, ed. Blake (Bristol: John Wright, 1894), 21.

19. While these symptoms are indeed rare today, the lawyer of a patient that had killed his wife and their two children on the account of being hypothyroid contacted me for a consultation. In another instance, a seemingly normal patient of mine developed delusions and was committed shortly after he stopped taking his daily treatment tablets.

20. Hospital de São José, a public hospital, serves the greater Lisbon area as part of the Central Lisbon University Hospital Centre (CHULC). It replaced the fifteenth-century All Saints' Royal Hospital, which was destroyed in the 1755 Lisbon earthquake. Hospital de São José was the country's greatest school of surgery. In 1825, King John VI created the Royal School of Surgery (Escola Régia de Cirurgia), which would later evolve into the Lisbon Medical-Surgical School.

21. S. Slater, "The Discovery of Thyroid Replacement Therapy: Part 3: A Complete Transformation," *Journal of the Royal Society of Medicine* 104, no. 3 (2011): 100–106, quotation on 102.

22. G. R. Murray, "Note on the Treatment of Myxoedema by Hypodermic Injections of an Extract of the Thyroid Gland of a Sheep," *British Medical Journal* 2, no. 1606 (1891): 796–97.

23. E. L. Fox, "A Case of Myxoedema Treated by Taking Extract of Thyroid by the Mouth," *British Medical Journal* 2, no. 1661 (1892): 941.

24. H. W. Mackenzie, "A Case of Myxoedema Treated with Great Benefit by Feeding with Fresh Thyroid Glands," *British Medical Journal* 2, no. 1661 (1892): 940–41.

25. Blake, "Myxedema."

26. A. S. Jackson, "Diagnosis and Treatment of Myxedema and Cretinism," in *Goiter and Other Diseases of the Thyroid Gland*, ed. Jackson (New York: Pail B. Hoeber, 1926), 131–49.

27. G. R. Murray, "Myxedema," in *Diseases of the Thyroid Gland*, ed. Murray (London: H. K. Lewis, 1900), chap. 6.

28. H. R. Harrower, *Practical Organotherapy* (Glendale: Harrower Laboratory, 1920).

29. Sun Simiao, a Chinese physician and writer of the Sui and Tang dynasty, is credited with recognizing in 652 AD that goiter could be treated with chopped-up thyroid glands from pig, deer, water buffalo, and sheep. Many other reports exist in the Chinese medical literature from around the same time of the use of chopped-up thyroid of the gelded ram, sucking on the juice of a sheep thyroid, and even air-drying various animal thyroids for a powder to be taken every night with wine.

30. See H. Richardson, *The Thyroid and Parathyroid Glands* (Philadelphia: P. Blakiston's Son, 1905).

31. J. H. Means, "Mixedema," in *The Thyroid and Its Diseases*, ed. Means (Philadelphia: J. B. Lippincott, 1937), 236.

32. Richardson, *The Thyroid and Parathyroid Glands*, 197.

33. Means, "Mixedema," 237.

34. See Richardson, *The Thyroid and Parathyroid Glands*, 196.

35. See Means, "Mixedema," 228–61.

36. See "Method of Treatment," in *The Thyroid and Its Diseases*, ed. L. J. DeGroot and J. B. Stanbury (New York: Wiley & Sons, 1975), 449.

37. See "Adult Hypothyroidism," in *The Thyroid and Its Diseases*, ed. L. J. DeGroot, P. R. Larsen, and G. Hennemann (New York: Churchill Livingstone, 1996), 351.

38. "Older Therapies Aren't Necessarily Better for Thyroid Hormone Replacement," US Food & Drug Administration, last updated June 14, 2021, https://www.fda.gov/consumers/consumer-updates/older-therapies-arent-necessarily-better-thyroid-hormone-replacement.

CHAPTER 7

1. C. R. Harington, *The Thyroid Gland* (London: Oxford University Press, 1933), 22–23.

2. E. Baumann, "Über das normale Vorkommen von Jod im Thierkorper," *Zeitschrift fur Physiologische Chemie* 21 (1896): 319.

3. J. C. Morris and V. A. Galton, "The Isolation of Thyroxine (T4), the Discovery of 3,5,3'-triiodothyronine (T3), and the Identification of the Deiodinases That Generate T3 from T4: An Historical Review," *Endocrine* 66, no. 1 (2019): 3–9.

4. Plummer was also one of the founding partners of the clinic, who for years made extended clinical studies of thyroid disturbances in several thousand cases of goiter. In 1928, he described a form of hyperthyroidism caused by thyroid nodules that to this day is known as Plummer's disease.

5. E. C. Kendall, "Reminiscences on the Isolation of Thyroxine," *Mayo Clinic Proceedings*, August 1964, 548–52.

6. A. Nürnberg, "Zur Kenntnis des Jodothyrins," *Hofmeisters Beiträge* 10 (1907): 125.

7. E. C. Kendall, *Thyroxine* (New York: Chemical Catalog, 1929), 24.

8. H. Himsworth and R. V. Pitt-Rivers, "Charles Robert Harington, 1897–1972," *Biographical Memoirs of Fellows of the Royal Society* 18 (1972): 267–308.

9. Harington, *The Thyroid Gland*, 94.

10. R. Pitt-Rivers, "Sir Charles Harington and the Structure of Thyroxine," *Mayo Clinic Proceedings*, August 1964, 553–59.

11. J. R. Tata, "Rosalind Venetia Pitt-Rivers, 4 March 1907–14 January 1990," *Biographical Memoirs of Fellows of the Royal Society* 39 (1994): 326–48.

12. B. W. Hart, *George Pitt-Rivers and the Nazis* (London: Bloomsbury Academic, 2015).

13. She studied at Bedford College, where she was awarded a bachelor of science in 1930 and a master of science in 1931. Despite the outbreak of war, and as a single mother, Pitt-Rivers chose to stay in London and worked at the blood bank, as she was determined to help in the war effort. During the Blitz of 1940, she got around London on a motorcycle. She refused to seek refuge in bomb shelters—she preferred to sleep in her bed.

14. See J. Gross and R. Pitt-Rivers, "The Identification of 3:5:3'-L-triiodothyronine in Human Plasma," *Lancet* 259, no. 6705 (1952): 439–41; J. Gross and R. Pitt-Rivers, "Physiological Activity of 3:5:3'-L-triiodothyronine," *Lancet* 259, no. 6708 (1952): 593–94; and J. Gross, R. Pitt-Rivers, and W. R. Trotter, "Effect of 3:5:3'-L-triiodothyronine in Myxoedema," *Lancet* 259, no. 6717 (1952):1044–45.

15. Tata, "Rosalind Venetia Pitt-Rivers."

CHAPTER 8

1. Braverman, Ingbar, and Sterling, "Conversion of Thyroxine (T4) to Triiodothyronine (T3)."

2. Taylor, Kapur, and Adie, "Combined Thyroxine and Triiodothyronine."

3. S. P. Asper Jr., H. A. Selenkow, and C. A. Plamondon, "A Comparison of the Metabolic Activities of 3,5,3-L-triiodothyronine and L-thyroxine in Myxedema," *Bulletin of the Johns Hopkins Hospital* 93, no. 3 (1953): 164–98.

4. Braverman, Ingbar, and Sterling, "Conversion of Thyroxine (T4) to Triiodothyronine (T3)."

5. J. Gross, and C. P. Leblond, "Metabolites of Thyroxine," *Proceedings of the Society for Experimental Biology and Medicine* 76, no. 4 (1951): 686–89.

6. E. C. Albright, F. C. Larson, and R. H. Tust, "In vitro Conversion of Thyroxin to Triiodothyronine by Kidney Slices," *Proceedings of the Society for Experimental Biology and Medicine* 86, no. 1 (1954): 137–40.

7. J. B. Stanbury, *The Iodine Trail* (Oxford: Oxford University Press, 2008).

8. R. Pitt-Rivers, J. B. Stanbury, and B. Rapp, "Conversion of Thyroxine to 3-5-3'-triiodothyronine in vivo," *Journal of Clinical Endocrinology and Metabolism* 15, no. 5 (1955): 616–20.

9. W. R. Lassiter and J. B. Stanbury, "The in vivo Conversion of Thyroxine to 3:5:3'triiodothyronine," *Journal of Clinical Endocrinology and Metabolism* 18, no. 8 (1958): 903–6.

10. Clark Sawin History Resource Center, "Thyroid History Timeline: 1962: Rosalind Pitt-Rivers Lecture," parts 1 and 2, American Thyroid Association, n.d.,

last accessed February 12, 2022, https://www.thyroid.org/about-american-thyroid-association/clark-t-sawin-history-resource-center/thyroid-history-timeline/.

11. Galton, Larsen, and Berry, "The Deiodinases: Their Identification and Cloning."

12. Braverman, Ingbar, and Sterling, "Conversion of Thyroxine (T4) to Triiodothyronine (T3)."

13. K. Sterling, M. A. Brenner, and E. S. Newman, "Conversion of Thyroxine to Triiodothyronine in Normal Human Subjects," *Science* 169, no. 3950 (1970): 1099–100. See also Braverman, Ingbar, and Sterling, "Conversion of Thyroxine (T4) to Triiodothyronine (T3)."

14. J. H. Oppenheimer and H. L. Schwartz, "Molecular Basis of Thyroid Hormone-Dependent Brain Development," *Endocrine Reviews* 18, no. 4 (1997): 462–75.

15. Taylor, Kapur, and Adie, "Combined Thyroxine and Triiodothyronine"; C. T. Sawin, W. P. Castelli, J. M. Hershman, P. McNamara, and P. Bacharach, "The Aging Thyroid: Thyroid Deficiency in the Framingham Study," *Archives of Internal Medicine* 145, no. 8 (1985): 1386–88.

CHAPTER 9

1. D. Carr, D. T. McLeod, G. Parry, and H. M. Thornes, "Fine Adjustment of Thyroxine Replacement Dosage: Comparison of the Thyrotrophin Releasing Hormone Test Using a Sensitive Thyrotrophin Assay with Measurement of Free Thyroid Hormones and Clinical Assessment," *Clinical Endocrinology* 28, no. 3 (1988): 325–33.

2. Roberts, "Psychological Problems in Thyroid Disease."

3. J. H. Lazarus, "Investigation and Treatment of Hypothyroidism," *Clinical Endocrinology* 44, no. 2 (1996): 129–31.

4. H. Zulewski, D. Muller, P. Daci, A. R. Miserez, and J. J. Staub, "Estimation of Tissue Hypothyroidism by a New Clinical Score: Evaluation of Patients with Various Grades of Hypothyroidism and Controls," *Journal of Clinical Endocrinology and Metabolism* 82, no. 3 (1997): 771–76.

5. Saravanan, Chau, Roberts, Vedhara, Greenwood, and Dayan, "Psychological Well-Being in Patients."

6. See Wekking, Appelhof, Fliers, et al., "Cognitive Functioning and Well-Being in Euthyroid Patients." The following paragraphs are sourced from this article.

7. M. H. Samuels, K. G. Schuff, N. E. Carlson, P. Carello, and J. S. Janowsky, "Health Status, Psychological Symptoms, Mood, and Cognition in L-thyroxine-Treated Hypothyroid Subjects," *Thyroid* 17, no. 3 (2007): 249–58.

8. H. J. Wouters, H. C. van Loon, M. M. van der Klauw, et al., "No Effect of the Thr92Ala Polymorphism of Deiodinase-2 on Thyroid Hormone Parameters, Health-Related Quality of Life, and Cognitive Functioning in a Large Population-Based Cohort Study," *Thyroid* 27, no. 2 (2017): 147–55.

9. See S. J. Peterson, E. A. McAninch, and A. C. Bianco, "Is a Normal TSH Syn-

onymous with 'Euthyroidism' in Levothyroxine Monotherapy?," *Journal of Clinical Endocrinology and Metabolism* 101, no. 12 (2016): jc20162660.

10. C. A. Gorman, N. S. Jiang, R. D. Ellefson, and L. R. Elveback, "Comparative Effectiveness of Dextrothyroxine and Levothyroxine in Correcting Hypothyroidism and Lowering Blood Lipid Levels in Hypothyroid Patients," *Journal of Clinical Endocrinology and Metabolism* 49, no. 1 (1979): 1–7.

11. Ridgway, Cooper, Walker, et al., "Therapy of Primary Hypothyroidism with L-triiodothyronine."

12. M. H. Samuels, I. Kolobova, A. Smeraglio, D. Peters, J. Q. Purnell, K. G. Schuff, "Effects of Levothyroxine Replacement or Suppressive Therapy on Energy Expenditure and Body Composition," *Thyroid* 26, no. 3 (2016): 347–55.

13. E. Muraca, S. Ciardullo, A. Oltolini, et al., "Resting Energy Expenditure in Obese Women with Primary Hypothyroidism and Appropriate Levothyroxine Replacement Therapy," *Journal of Clinical Endocrinology and Metabolism* 105, no. 4 (2020).

14. J. P. Werneck de Castro, T. L. Fonseca, C. B. Ueta, et al., "Differences in Hypothalamic Type 2 Deiodinase Ubiquitination Explain Localized Sensitivity to Thyroxine," *Journal of Clinical Investigation* 125, no. 2 (2015): 769–81.

15. Y. K. Lee, H. Lee, S. Han, et al., "Association between Thyroid-Stimulating Hormone Level after Total Thyroidectomy and Hypercholesterolemia in Female Patients with Differentiated Thyroid Cancer: A Retrospective Study," *Journal of Clinical Medicine* 8, no. 8 (2019); M. Ito, A Miyauchi, M Hisakado, et al., "Biochemical Markers Reflecting Thyroid Function in Athyreotic Patients on Levothyroxine Monotherapy," *Thyroid* 27, no. 4 (2017): 484–90.

16. E. A. McAninch, K. B. Rajan, C. H. Miller, and A. C. Bianco, "Systemic Thyroid Hormone Status during Levothyroxine Therapy in Hypothyroidism: A Systematic Review and Meta-analysis," *Journal of Clinical Endocrinology and Metabolism* 103, no. 12 (2018): 4533–42.

17. Peterson, McAninch, and Bianco, "Is a Normal TSH Synonymous with 'Euthyroidism'?"

18. T. Idrees, W. H. Prieto, S. Casula, et al., "Use of Statins among Patients Taking Levothyroxine: An Observational Drug Utilization Study Across Sites," *Journal of the Endocrine Society* 5, no. 7 (2021): bvab038.

CHAPTER 10

1. See E. Silva, "Disposal Rates of Thyroxine and Triiodothyronine in Iodine-Deficient Rats," *Endocrinology* 91, no. 6 (1972): 1430–35; and G. M. Abrams and P. R. Larsen, "Triiodothyronine and Thyroxine in the Serum and Thyroid Glands of Iodine-Deficient Rats," *Journal of Clinical Investigation* 52 (1973): 2522–31.

2. P. R. Larsen, "Thyroid-Pituitary Interaction: Feedback Regulation of Thyrotropin Secretion by Thyroid Hormones," *New England Journal of Medicine* 306, no. 1 (1982): 23–32.

3. D. L. Geffner, M. Azukizawa, and J. M. Hershman, "Propylthiouracil Blocks Extrathyroidal Conversion of Thyroxine to Triiodothyronine and Augments Thyrotropin Secretion in Man," *Journal of Clinical Investigation* 55, no. 2 (1975): 224–49.

4. D. L. St. Germain, "The Effects and Interactions of Substrates, Inhibitors, and the Cellular Thiol-disulfide Balance on the Regulation of Type II Iodothyronine 5'-deiodinase," *Endocrinology* 122, no. 5 (1988): 1860–68.

5. St. Germain, "Effects and Interactions of Substrates, Inhibitors."

6. J. L. Leonard, C. A. Siegrist-Kaiser, and C. J. Zuckerman, "Regulation of Type II Iodothyronine 5'-deiodinase by Thyroid Hormone: Inhibition of Actin Polymerization Blocks Enzyme Inactivation in cAMP-Stimulated Glial Cells," *Journal of Biological Chemistry* 265, no. 2 (1990): 940–46.

7. J. Steinsapir, J. Harney, and P. R. Larsen, "Type 2 Iodothyronine Deiodinase in Rat Pituitary Tumor Cells Is Inactivated in Proteasomes," *Journal of Clinical Investigation* 102, no. 11 (1998): 1895–99.

8. B. Gereben, C. Goncalves, J. W. Harney, P. R. Larsen, and A. C. Bianco, "Selective Proteolysis of Human Type 2 Deiodinase: A Novel Ubiquitin-Proteasomal Mediated Mechanism for Regulation of Hormone Activation," *Molecular Endocrinology* 14, no. 11 (2000): 1697–708.

9. Callebaut, Curcio-Morelli, Mornon, et al., "Iodothyronine Selenodeiodinases Are Thioredoxin-Fold Family Proteins."

10. M. Dentice, A. Bandyopadhyay, B. Gereben, et al., "The Hedgehog-Inducible Ubiquitin Ligase Subunit WSB-1 Modulates Thyroid Hormone Activation and PTHrP Secretion in the Developing Growth Plate," *Nature Cell Biology* 7, no. 7 (2005): 698–705.

11. C. Curcio-Morelli, A. M. Zavacki, M. Christofollete, et al., "Deubiquitination of Type 2 Iodothyronine Deiodinase by von Hippel–Lindau Protein-Interacting Deubiquitinating Enzymes Regulates Thyroid Hormone Activation," *Journal of Clinical Investigation* 112, no. 2 (2003): 189–96.

12. Werneck de Castro, Fonseca, Ueta, et al., "Differences in Hypothalamic Type 2 Deiodinase Ubiquitination."

13. See C. Fekete, B. C. Freitas, A. Zeold, et al., "Expression Patterns of WSB-1 and USP-33 Underlie Cell-Specific Posttranslational Control of Type 2 Deiodinase in the Rat Brain," *Endocrinology* 148, no. 10 (2007): 4865–74.

14. See Werneck de Castro, Fonseca, Ueta, et al., "Differences in Hypothalamic Type 2 Deiodinase Ubiquitination."

CHAPTER 11

1. See Stock, Surks, and Oppenheimer, "Replacement Dosage of L-thyroxine in Hypothyroidism."

2. C. T. Sawin, J. M. Hershman, R. Fernandez-Garcia, S. Ghazvinian, O. P. Ganda, and M. Azukizawa, "A Comparison of Thyroxine and Desicatted Thyroid in Patients with Primary Hypothyroidism," *Metabolism* 27, no. 10 (1978): 1518–25.

3. See Ingbar, Borges, Iflah, Kleinmann, Braverman, and Ingbar, "Elevated Serum Thyroxine Concentration."

4. See Gross and Pitt-Rivers, "Identification of 3:5:3'-L-triiodothyronine"; and Gross and Pitt-Rivers, "Physiological Activity of 3:5:3'-L-triiodothyronine."

5. W. Croteau, J. C. Davey, V. A. Galton, and D. L. St. Germain, "Cloning of the Mammalian Type II Iodothyronine Deiodinase: A Selenoprotein Differentially Expressed and Regulated in Human and Rat Brain and Other Tissues," *Journal of Clinical Investigation* 98, no. 2 (1996): 405-17.

6. M. J. Schneider, S. N. Fiering, S. E. Pallud, A. F. Parlow, D. L. St. Germain, and V. A. Galton, "Targeted Disruption of the Type 2 Selenodeiodinase Gene (DIO2) Results in a Phenotype of Pituitary Resistance to T4," *Molecular Endocrinology* 15, no. 12 (2001): 2137-48.

7. M. A. Christoffolete, R. Arrojo e Drigo, F. Gazoni, et al., "Mice with Impaired Extrathyroidal Thyroxine to 3,5,3'-triiodothyronine Conversion Maintain Normal Serum 3,5,3'-triiodothyronine Concentrations," *Endocrinology* 148, no. 3 (2007): 954-60.

8. See Stock, Surks, and Oppenheimer, "Replacement Dosage of L-thyroxine in Hypothyroidism"; Ingbar, Borges, Iflah, Kleinmann, Braverman, and Ingbar, "Elevated Serum Thyroxine Concentration"; and Sawin, Hershman, Fernandez-Garcia, Ghazvinian, Ganda, and Azukizawa, "A Comparison of Thyroxine and Desicatted Thyroid."

9. See D. Gullo, A. Latina, F. Frasca, R. Le Moli, G. Pellegriti, and R. Vigneri, "Levothyroxine Monotherapy Cannot Guarantee Euthyroidism in All Athyreotic Patients," *PLOS One* 6, no. 8 (2011): e22552; Ridgway, Cooper, Walker, et al., "Therapy of Primary Hypothyroidism with L-triiodothyronine"; Kahn, "Serum Triiodothyronine Levels"; Murchison, Chesters, and Bewsher, "Serum Thyroid Hormone Levels"; Salmon, Rendell, Williams, et al., "Chemical Hyperthyroidism"; and Erfurth and Hedner, "Thyroid Hormone Metabolism in Thyroid Disease."

10. See J. Jonklaas, B. Davidson, S. Bhagat, and S. J. Soldin, "Triiodothyronine Levels in Athyreotic Individuals during Levothyroxine Therapy," *JAMA* 299, no. 7 (2008): 769-77; Jennings, O'Malley, Griffin, Northover, and Rosenthal, "Relevance of Increased Serum Thyroxine Concentrations"; Pearce and Himsworth, "Total and Free Thyroid Hormone Concentrations"; Fish, Schwartz, Cavanaugh, Steffes, Bantle, and Oppenheimer, "Replacement Dose, Metabolism, and Bioavailability of Levothyroxine"; and Samuels, Schuff, Carlson, Carello, and Janowsky, "Health Status, Psychological Symptoms, Mood."

11. Gullo, Latina, Frasca, Le Moli, Pellegriti, and Vigneri, "Levothyroxine Monotherapy Cannot Guarantee Euthyroidism."

12. Peterson, McAninch, and Bianco, "Is a Normal TSH Synonymous with 'Euthyroidism'?"

13. B. M. Bocco, J. P. Werneck-de-Castro, K. C. Oliveira, et al., "Type 2 Deiodinase Disruption in Astrocytes Results in Anxiety-Depressive-Like Behavior in Male Mice," *Endocrinology* 157, no. 9 (2016): 3682-95.

14. Ridgway, Cooper, Walker, et al., "Therapy of Primary Hypothyroidism with L-triiodothyronine."

15. Ridgway, Cooper, Walker, et al.

16. For the guidelines, see Singer, Cooper, Levy, et al., "Treatment Guidelines for Patients." For the studies, see above, n8-10.

17. See Garber, Cobin, Gharib, et al., "Clinical Practice Guidelines for Hypothyroidism in Adults"; and Jonklaas, Davidson, Bhagat, and Soldin, "Triiodothyronine Levels in Athyreotic Individuals."

18. Stock, Surks, and Oppenheimer, "Replacement Dosage of L-thyroxine in Hypothyroidism"; Ingbar, Borges, Iflah, Kleinmann, Braverman, and Ingbar, "Elevated Serum Thyroxine Concentration"; Ridgway, Cooper, Walker, et al., "Therapy of Primary Hypothyroidism with L-triiodothyronine"; Kahn, "Serum Triiodothyronine Levels"; Murchison, Chesters, and Bewsher, "Serum Thyroid Hormone Levels"; Salmon, Rendell, Williams, et al., "Chemical Hyperthyroidism"; Erfurth and Hedner, "Thyroid Hormone Metabolism in Thyroid Disease"; Gullo, Latina, Frasca, Le Moli, Pellegriti, and Vigneri, "Levothyroxine Monotherapy Cannot Guarantee Euthyroidism."

19. See Gullo, Latina, Frasca, Le Moli, Pellegriti, and Vigneri, "Levothyroxine Monotherapy Cannot Guarantee Euthyroidism."

CHAPTER 12

1. M. D. Ettleson and A. C. Bianco, "Individualized Therapy for Hypothyroidism: Is T4 Enough for Everyone?," *Journal of Clinical Endocrinology and Metabolism* 105, no. 9 (2020).

2. D. Mentuccia, L. Proietti-Pannunzi, K. Tanner, et al., "Association between a Novel Variant of the Human Type 2 Deiodinase Gene Thr92Ala and Insulin Resistance: Evidence of Interaction with the Trp64Arg Variant of the Beta-3-adrenergic Receptor," *Diabetes* 51, no. 3 (2002): 880–83.

3. Callebaut, Curcio-Morelli, Mornon, et al., "Iodothyronine Selenodeiodinases Are Thioredoxin-Fold Family Proteins."

4. See V. Panicker, P. Saravanan, B. Vaidya, et al., "Common Variation in the DIO2 Gene Predicts Baseline Psychological Well-Being and Response to Combination Thyroxine plus Triiodothyronine Therapy in Hypothyroid Patients," *Journal of Clinical Endocrinology and Metabolism* 94, no. 5 (2009): 1623–29.

5. Jo, Fonseca, Bocco, et al., "Type 2 Deiodinase Polymorphism."

6. Castagna, Dentice, Cantara, et al., "DIO2 Thr92Ala Reduces Deiodinase-2 Activity."

7. Jo, Fonseca, Bocco, et al., "Type 2 Deiodinase Polymorphism."

8. E. A. McAninch, S. Jo, N. Z. Preite, et al., "Prevalent Polymorphism in Thyroid Hormone-Activating Enzyme Leaves a Genetic fingerprint that underlies associated clinical syndromes," *Journal of Clinical Endocrinology and Metabolism* 100, no. 3 (2015): 920–33.

9. McAninch, Jo, Preite, et al., "Prevalent Polymorphism in Thyroid Hormone-Activating Enzyme."

10. McAninch, Jo, Preite, et al.

11. E. A. McAninch, K. B. Rajan, D. A. Evans, et al., "A Common DIO2 Polymorphism and Alzheimer Disease Dementia in African and European Americans," *Journal of Clinical Endocrinology and Metabolism* 103, no. 5 (2018): 1818–26.

12. A. C. Bianco and B. S. Kim, "Pathophysiological Relevance of Deiodinase Polymorphism," *Current Opinion in Endocrinology, Diabetes, and Obesity* 25, no. 5 (2018): 341–46.

13. R. P. Peeters, H. van Toor, W. Klootwijk, et al., "Polymorphisms in Thyroid Hormone Pathway Genes Are Associated with Plasma TSH and Iodothyronine Levels in Healthy Subjects," *Journal of Clinical Endocrinology and Metabolism* 88, no. 6 (2003): 2880–88.

14. Franca, German, Fernandes, et al., "Human Type 1 Iodothyronine Deiodinase (DIO1) Mutations."

15. H. K. Nayak, M. K. Daga, R. Kumar, S. K. Garg, N. Kumar, P. K. Mohanty, "A Series Report of Autoimmune Hypothyroidism Associated with Hashimoto's Encephalopathy: An Under Diagnosed Clinical Entity with Good Prognosis," *BMJ Case Reports* (2010).

16. K. Müssig, T. Leyhe, S. Holzmüller, et al., "Increased Prevalence of Antibodies to Central Nervous System Tissue and Gangliosides in Hashimoto's Thyroiditis Compared to Other Thyroid Illnesses," *Psychoneuroendocrinology* 34, no. 8 (2009): 1252–56.

17. G. Zettinig, S. Asenbaum, B. J. Fueger, et al., "Increased Prevalence of Subclinical Brain Perfusion Abnormalities in Patients with Autoimmune Thyroiditis: Evidence of Hashimoto's Encephalitis?," *Clinical Endocrinology* 59, no. 5 (2003): 637–43.

18. J. Bladowska, M. Waliszewska-Prosól, M. Ejma, and M. Sąsiadek, "The Metabolic Alterations within the Normal Appearing Brain in Patients with Hashimoto's Thyroiditis Are Correlated with Hormonal Changes," *Metabolic Brain Disease* 34, no. 1 (2019): 53–60.

19. R. Green, L. H. Allen, A. L. Bjørke-Monsen, et al., "Vitamin B(12) Deficiency," *Nature Reviews Disease Primers* 3 (2017): 17040.

20. A. B. Collins and R. Pawlak, "Prevalence of Vitamin B-12 Deficiency among Patients with Thyroid Dysfunction," *Asia Pacific Journal of Clinical Nutrition* 25, no. 2 (2016): 221–26.

CHAPTER 13

1. See J. M. Millan-Alanis, J. G. Gonzalez-Gonzalez, A. Flores-Rodríguez, et al., "Benefits and Harms of Levothyroxine/Liothyronine vs. Levothyroxine Monotherapy for Adult Patients with Hypothyroidism: Systematic Review and Meta-analysis," *Thyroid* (August 2021). The following paragraphs are sourced from this article.

2. See G. P. Leese, E. Soto-Pedre, and L. A. Donnelly, "Liothyronine Use in a 17 Year Observational Population-Based Study—the Tears Study," *Clinical Endocrinology* 85, no. 6 (2016): 918–25; and T. Planck, F. Hedberg, J. Calissendorff, and A. Nilsson, "Liothyronine Use in Hypothyroidism and Its Effects on Cancer and Mortality," *Thyroid* 31, no. 5 (2021): 732–39.

3. Idrees, Palmer, Maciel, and Bianco, "Liothyronine and Desiccated Thyroid Extract."

4. See, for example, E. Diener, "Subjective Well-Being: The Science of Happiness and a Proposal for a National Index," *American Psychologist* 55 (2000): 34-43; T. Hartig, M. Mang, and G. W. Evans, "Restorative Effects of Natural Environment Experiences," *Environment and Behavior* 23, no. 1 (1991): 3–26; and A. E. Van Den Berg, T. Hartig, and H. Staats, "Preference for Nature in Urbanized Societies: Stress, Restoration, and the Pursuit of Sustainability," *Journal of Social Issues* 63, no. 1 (2007): 79–96.

CHAPTER 14

1. See Jonklaas, Bianco, Bauer, et al., "Guidelines for the Treatment of Hypothyroidism."

2. See Peterson, Cappola, Castro, et al., "Online Survey of Hypothyroid Patients."

3. See J. Jonklaas, E. Tefera, and N. Shara, "Prescribing Therapy for Hypothyroidism: Influence of Physician Characteristics," *Thyroid* 29, no. 1 (2019): 44–52; J. Jonklaas, E. Tefera, and N. Shara, "Short-Term Time Trends in Prescribing Therapy for Hypothyroidism: Results of a Survey of American Thyroid Association Members," *Frontiers in Endocrinology (Lausanne)* 10 (2019): 31; and J. Jonklaas, E. Tefera, and N. Shara, "Physician Choice of Hypothyroidism Therapy: Influence of Patient Characteristics," *Thyroid* 28, no. 11 (2018): 1416–24.

4. See J. Jonklaas, A. C. Bianco, A. R. Cappola, et al., "Evidence-Based Use of Levothyroxine/Liothyronine Combinations in Treating Hypothyroidism: A Consensus Document," *Thyroid* 31, no. 2 (2021): 156–82.

5. M. K. M. Shakir, D. I. Brooks, E. A. McAninch, et al., "Comparative Effectiveness of Levothyroxine, Desiccated Thyroid Extract, and Levothyroxine + Liothyronine in Hypothyroidism," *Journal of Clinical Endocrinology and Metabolism* 106, no. 11 (2021): e4400–4413.

6. Shakir, Brooks, McAninch, et al., "Comparative Effectiveness of Levothyroxine, Thyroid Extract, and Levothyroxine + Liothyronine."

7. See W. M. Wiersinga, "T4 + T3 Combination Therapy: Any Progress?," *Endocrine* 66, no. 1 (2019): 70–78.

8. See B. Van Tassell, G. F. Wohlford IV, J. D. Linderman, et al., "Pharmacokinetics of L-triiodothyronine in Patients Undergoing Thyroid Hormone Therapy Withdrawal," *Thyroid* 29, no. 10 (2019): 1371–79.

9. B. B. Medici, J. L. la Cour, L. F. Michaelsson, J. O. Faber, and B. Nygaard, "Nei-

ther Baseline nor Changes in Serum Triiodothyronine during Levothyroxine/Liothyronine Combination Therapy Predict a Positive Response to This Treatment Modality in Hypothyroid Patients with Persistent Symptoms," *European Thyroid Journal* 6, no. 2 (2017): 89–93.

10. S. Reddy, "New Call for More Thyroid Options," *Wall Street Journal*, August 5, 2013.

CHAPTER 15

1. Jonklaas, Bianco, Bauer, et al., "Guidelines for the Treatment of Hypothyroidism."

2. E. Roti, R. Minelli, E. Gardini, and L. E. Braverman, "The Use and Misuse of Thyroid Hormone," *Endocrine Reviews* 14, no. 4 (1993): 401–23.

3. T. Idrees, J. D. Price, T. Piccariello, and A. C. Bianco, "Sustained Release T3 Therapy: Animal Models and Translational Applications," *Frontiers in Endocrinology (Lausanne)* (August 13, 2019), https://doi.org/10.3389/fendo.2019.00544.

4. G. Hennemann, R. Docter, T. J. Visser, P. T. Postema, and E. P. Krenning, "Thyroxine plus Low-Dose, Slow-Release Triiodothyronine Replacement in Hypothyroidism: Proof of Principle," *Thyroid* 14, no. 4 (2004): 271–75.

5. F. Santini, G. Ceccarini, C. Pelosini, et al., "Treatment of Hypothyroid Patients with L-thyroxine (L-T4) plus Triiodothyronine Sulfate (T3S): A Phase II, Open-Label, Single Center, Parallel Groups Study on Therapeutic Efficacy and Tolerability," *Frontiers in Endocrinology (Lausanne)* 10 (2019): 826; F. Santini, M. Giannetti, I. Ricco, et al., "Steady-State Serum T3 Concentrations for 48 Hours Following the Oral Administration of a Single Dose of 3,5,3'-Triiodothyronine Sulfate (T3S)," *Endocrine Practice* 20, no. 7 (2014): 1–25; F. Santini, R. E. Hurd, B. Lee, and I. J. Chopra, "Thyromimetic Effects of 3,5,3'-triiodothyronine Sulfate in Hypothyroid Rats," *Endocrinology* 133, no. 1 (1993): 105–10.

6. R. R. Da Conceicao, G. W. Fernandes, T. L. Fonseca, B. Bocco, and A. C. Bianco, "Metal Coordinated Poly-zinc-liothyronine Provides Stable Circulating Triiodothyronine Levels in Hypothyroid Rats," *Thyroid* 28, no. 11 (2018): 1425–33.

7. R. R. Da Conceicao, G. W. Fernandes, T. L. Fonseca, B. Bocco, and A. C. Bianco, "Metal Coordinated Poly-zinc-liothyronine in Hypothyroid Rats."

8. R. R. Da Conceicao, G. W. Fernandes, T. L. Fonseca, B. Bocco, and A. C. Bianco, "Metal Coordinated Poly-zinc-liothyronine in Hypothyroid Rats."

9. A. M. Dumitrescu, E. C. Hanlon, M. Arosemena, et al., "Extended Absorption of Liothyronine from Poly-zinc-liothyronine [PZL]: Results from a Phase 1, Double-Blind, Randomized, and Controlled Study in Humans," *Thyroid* (2022), https://doi.org/10.1089/thy.2021.3034.

10. F. Santini, P. Vitti, L. Chiovato, et al., "Role for Inner Ring Deiodination Pre-

venting Transcutaneous Passage of Thyroxine," *Journal of Clinical Endocrinology and Metabolism* 88, no. 6 (2003): 2825–30.

11. See F. Antonica, D. F. Kasprzyk, R. Opitz, et al., "Generation of Functional Thyroid from Embryonic Stem Cells," *Nature* 491, no. 7422 (2012): 66–71.

12. See A. A. Kurmann, M. Serra, F. Hawkins, et al., "Regeneration of Thyroid Function by Transplantation of Differentiated Pluripotent Stem Cells," *Cell Stem Cell* 17, no. 5 (2015): 527–42.

13. See R. Latif, R. Ma, S. A. Morshed, B. Tokat, and T. F. Davies, "Long Term Rescue of the TSH Receptor Knock-Out Mouse—Thyroid Stem Cell Transplantation Restores Thyroid Function," *Frontiers in Endocrinology (Lausanne)* (2021): https://doi.org/10.3389/fendo.2021.706101.

EPILOGUE

1. Ireland, *Cretinism*, 244.

INDEX

University of Miami clinic, 9, 23–30, 150, 156, 166, 204, 239, 255
University of Minnesota, 130
University of Naples, 177, 202
University of Pisa, 244
University of São Paulo, 92–93
University of Wisconsin, 144
untested treatments: blood and, 138–41, 145–46, 149, 151; brain and, 150; children and, 148; clinical trials and, 143, 150; combination therapy and, 143, 150; dangers of, 137–51; diagnostics and, 137–39; dogma and, 151; endocrinology and, 139, 144–48; fatigue and, 151; FDA and, 143; goiter and, 144–45; Gross and, 143–47; heart and, 137; hormones and, 138–42, 145–46, 149, 151; iodine and, 141, 144–45, 148–49; Larsen and, 141, 144; liotrix, 123, 142–43; memory and, 150; metabolism and, 141–42, 147; Pitt-Rivers and, 143, 145, 147; prescriptions and, 151; quality of life and, 150; supplementation therapy and, 112, 122; Synthroid, 138, 147; T_3 and, 138–51; T_4 and, 138–51, T_4–T_3 transformation and, 143; thyroid extract and, 137–43, 149–50; TSH and, 137–43, 150–51; weight and, 150
USDA, 124
Utiger, Robert D., 138–39

Van Tassell, B., 237
Victoria, Queen, 112
Virginia Commonwealth University, 199
vision, 9
vitamins, 4, 29, 196, 210, 225

Wales, 21, 70, 110, 112, 155, 156–57
Wall Street Journal, 50–53, 58–59
Walter Reed National Military Medical Center, 232–33
weight: calories and, 2, 163–64; combination therapy and, 216–17; fatigue and, 2–3, 14, 29; gaining, 2–3, 9, 11, 14, 28–29, 150, 162, 164, 166, 200, 217; loss of, 36, 127; obesity, 127, 165, 201; quality of life and, 162–66; T_3, missed clues and, 190, 193; T_3 levels and, 200; thyroid extract and, 124; TSH and, 29, 64, 150, 166, 178; untested treatments and, 150
Wekking, Ellie, 159
Werneck, João Pedro, 34–35
Wharton, Thomas, 1–2
Wiersinga, Wilmar, 158–59, 236–37
women: Brigham and Women's Hospital, 88, 93, 98, 101, 170; guidelines and, 70; hypothyroidism susceptibility of, 6; iodine and, 80, 83; nineteenth-century treatments and, 109, 112–13; openness to alternative approaches, 232, 235; pharmaceutical companies and, 50; pregnancy and, 2 (see also pregnancy); quality of life and, 165, 167; surveys of, 14; T_4 and, 6, 26, 30, 50, 70, 88, 165, 167, 170, 235; TSH and, 170
Wool, Marvin S., 142–43
World War II, 132–33, 144

Yalow, Rosalyn, 139
Yamanaka, Shinya, 251